THE PAPYRUS EBERS

ANCIENT EGYPTIAN MEDICINE
THE PAPYRUS EBERS

Translated from the German Version

By

CYRIL P. BRYAN

M.B., B.CH., B.A.O.

Demonstrator in Anatomy, University College, London

With an Introduction by

PROFESSOR G. ELLIOT SMITH

M.D., D.SC., LITT.D., F.R.C.P., F.R.S.

Professor of Anatomy, University College, London

ARES PUBLISHERS INC.

CHICAGO MCMLXXIV

Unchanged Reprint of the Edition:
London, 1930.
ARES PUBLISHERS INC.
150 E. Huron Street
Chicago, Illinois 60611
Printed in the United States of America
International Standard Book Number:
0-89005-004-X
Library of Congress Catalog Card Number:
74-77905

Those about to study Medicine, and the younger Physicians, should light their torches at the fires of the Ancients.

ROKITANSKY

TO

AIDAN:

MY BROTHER

CONTENTS

LIST OF ILLUSTRATIONS

INTRODUCTION

It is often assumed even by the most learned historians that the history of medicine began with the Greeks, and that before the time of Hippocrates there was little or nothing that can be called a science of medicine. Yet for more than thirty centuries before the emancipation of human reason in Ionia, numerous practitioners had been attempting to diagnose and treat disease in Egypt, Mesopotamia, and elsewhere.

The Papyrus Ebers is the longest and the most famous of the documents relating to this more ancient practice of medicine. The Papyrus, although written about 1500 B.C., is really a collection of bits and pieces of folk-lore, much of it five and some of it probably twenty centuries older. It is expressed in archaic phraseology, so that many of the terms relating to the diseases and drugs are impossible to identify. In the face of these insuperable difficulties, it is not surprising that most scholars have refrained from risking their reputation for scholarship by pretending to translate a technical document in which many of the technical terms are at present untranslatable.

An heroic attempt to provide a translation in German was made, however, many years ago by Dr. H. Joachim. This attempt naturally provoked many criticisms, especially from those scholars who had the philological knowledge to recognize the solecisms. But if the time is not yet ripe for an adequate translation, the Papyrus is so interesting that no excuse should be necessary for providing a rendering in English of the only version at present available for those who cannot read the scripts of Ancient Egypt. Hence Dr. Cyril Bryan is to be commended for giving us in English an interpretation based upon Dr. Joachim's translation, though not slavishly following it.

In his book, *Magician and Leech* (1929), Mr. Warren R. Dawson has given a very useful summary of the history of the various sources of our information concerning ancient medicine, with particular reference to the series of ancient Egyptian papyri. Concerning the Ebers Papyrus he writes :

'The Ebers Papyrus is the longest and most famous of these documents. It was found in a tomb at Thebes together with another medical text, the Edwin Smith Papyrus, about 1862, and was acquired by the Egyptologist whose name it bears. It is now preserved in the University of Leipzig, and is in almost perfect condition. The contents are medical and magical throughout, except that on the back of the manuscript is written a calendar which has been of the utmost importance in studying the difficult and complicated problems of Egyptian chronology. The Ebers Papyrus was written about 1500 B.C., but there is abundant evidence on philological and other grounds that it was copied from a series of books many centuries older. It is stated in the Papyrus itself that one passage dates from the First Dynasty (*circa* 3400 B.C.), and another extract is associated with a queen of the Sixth Dynasty. Such statements as these are of no positive value in dating, because it was in Egypt, as elsewhere, a common literary artifice to ascribe to books a very ancient origin in order to enhance their value and authority. Fortunately, however, there is no need to rely on such statements for dating Egyptian documents. Our knowledge of the writing, grammar and palæography of the papyri enables us to place them fairly accurately. Probably the books from which the Ebers Papyrus contains excerpts were written during the Twelfth and Thirteenth Dynasties, although it is likely that their subject-matter is many centuries older.

'The Ebers Papyrus is not a book in the proper sense of the word : it is a miscellaneous collection of extracts and jottings collected from at least forty different sources. It consists mainly of a large collection of prescriptions for a number of named ailments, specifying the names of the drugs, the quantities of each, and the method of administration. A few sections deal with diagnosis and symptoms, another passage is physiological in character and describes the action of the heart and its vessels, and the concluding portion is surgical, being concerned with the treatment of wounds and suppurating sores. Freely interspersed amongst these elements are spells and incantations. The text covers 110 large columns (each of 22 lines on the average) in the original roll, which a modern editor has conveniently divided into 877 numbered sections of varying length. 'In considering the pathology of the papyri, the student is at once confronted with a host of difficulties. In the first place, the texts are full of philological and lexicographical problems, and they are written in a specialized, concise and aphoristic style abounding in syntactical difficulties. Many of the passages, as already noted, have been copied from older books and show evidence of textual corruption. But the greatest difficulty of all is the impossibility of translating into English the names of a great number of the maladies mentioned, and the names of most of the drugs.'

In the identification of the diseases with which the ancient physicians were trying to cope, and of the drugs and other measures they were using for therapeutic purposes, the study of folk-lore, both of the Egyptians and other people, and the survival of ancient remedies, opens up great possibilities. It is the aim of Dr. Bryan's book to disseminate such information of ancient Egyptian medicine as we have and in particular to reveal the lacunæ in our knowledge. For our hope of gaining a fuller insight into the real meaning of these cryptic papyri depends largely upon the evidence which investigators of departments of learning other than Egyptian philology can provide. This book will provide students of folk-lore with many hints of help they may be able to give. How fruitful the use of the data of modern folk-lore can be in the study of the ancient Egyptian writings has been shown by Mr. Dawson in a number of memoirs which he has published. In this connection it is important not to forget that although the merits of many of the ancient materials used in the most ancient pharmacopœias are entirely illusory, at the same time the Egyptians did discover not a few substances whose virtues are recognized to-day as being quite genuine. For example many centuries before the Ebers Papyrus was written, the Egyptians had discovered and were using Castor Oil; they had recognized certain antiseptic virtues in Onions; and their belief in the virtues of a good many other substances, vegetable, animal, and mineral, which they used, has been shown to have a large measure of justification.

Another source of information has recently been tapped and promises to refresh a department of archæology which was threatened with sterility. It adds enormously to the interest and importance of such documents as the Ebers Papyrus and also provides a new and fruitful method for interpreting them. In his treatise *Die Sprache des Pentateuch in Ihren Beziehungen zum Ægyptischen*, Professor Λ. S. Yahouda has recently emphasized the extent to which the earlier parts of the Old Testament—and the medical lore it contains—was inspired by Egypt. Both in language and subject-matter the Five Books of Moses reveal the intimacy of the Egyptian influence, and he concludes that contrary to modern ideas the Pentateuch could have been compiled only at the time of the Exodus, when the writer's mind was saturated with the language and ideas of Ancient Egypt. Moses himself was 'the Child of the Nile' and the medical information in the Old Testament is essentially identical with that of the Ebers Papyrus.

A great deal of the discussion which has taken place with regard to ancient medicine and in particular with what is recorded in Egyptian papyri has been concerned with the contrast between Rational Medicine and Magic ; and no little obscurity has been introduced into the interpretation of the ancient practice of medicine as a result of these discussions. Hence it is worth while to refer briefly to the essential points at issue.

Obviously to a primitive people lacking in any accumulated knowledge or understanding of disease, the ailments of the body fall into two clearly defined groups. These were in the first place the injuries to the body and such obvious material facts as boils, ulcers, and other diseased conditions which could be detected by sight ; and there was the other group of subtle mysterious disturbances, concerning the cause of many of which, even to-day, we are ignorant—just as we are ignorant of the reasons underlying the manner in which the disturbance of health manifests itself in certain definite symptoms. In early times, however, such constitutional diseases, of which no obvious cause could be found, were regarded as an interference with the life process—some condition which imperilled the existence of life in the body and for which the rational treatment was the addition to the vital substance of something which would increase its quantity and so avert the peril to existence. The point that I specially want to emphasize is the fact that there was originally no conflict between the rational and the magical—that the things we call magical to-day were originally inspired by rational considerations, for which the people who originally invented these devices believed they had valid reasons for putting faith in them. Just as the early people believed that as blood was the substance of life and that the virtue in blood depended upon its redness, so that the red colour and any red substance could protect the body from the risk of death, so a vast number of other materials, ideas, and even words, acquired the merit of being life-giving, and therefore were rational means of treating any condition which seemed to imperil life, in other words, to remove the vital elements from the body.

But it may be protested that many of the therapeutic measures adopted in the Ebers Papyrus are not simply drugs which had acquired a reputation for which there was no adequate justification, but were in the nature of spells and incantations. Nevertheless, these different rites which Dr. Alan Gardiner has distinguished as 'manual' and 'oral'—the doing something with the hands or saying something with the mouth to cure disease—were clearly inspired in the beginning by rational considerations. In the beginning there was no distinction whatever between science and religion, or between magic and reason. As knowledge grew the wise men of the time formulated certain general theories of knowledge, and they applied the principles so enunciated to include all sorts of other applications of the general principle which were not originally included in that principle when it was first formulated. Hence all sorts of devices became drawn within the ambit of the generalization because to those learned in the traditions of their system such applications of the general principle seemed to be rational and justifiable. But when the validity of the general principle was destroyed, the practice, which had acquired a certain hold on the imagination as the result of long use, would tend to persist as a cherished belief long after any scientific justification for it had been destroyed.

For example, in a Predynastic cemetery in Upper Egypt I discovered in the stomachs of small children who had died nearly sixty centuries ago the remains of mice which had been skinned and eaten just before their death. (An account of the finding of this interesting material is given in my book, *The Ancient Egyptians.*) There is reason to believe that the faith in the mouse as a life-giving substance was due to the fact that after the inundation, when the mud left by the falling river became dried by the rays of the sun and mice were seen to emerge from these cracks, the Egyptians of sixty centuries ago believed, as their modern representatives believe to-day, that these mice were actually formed from the mud deposited by the river and that they represented the very quintessence of the life-giving virtues of the river itself—the life that manifested itself year by year in the barley which provided food for human beings, and from which, according to their traditions, the bodies and the very life of the men themselves were also formed. Hence these mice were regarded as one of the most potent elixirs of life, and therefore appropriate remedies for saving life under desperate circumstances. Learned men have known for several thousands of years that there is no justification for this belief in the virtues of mice as a drug, and yet it has persisted through the ages and is surreptitiously practised in England at the present day by thousands of people who have not the least suspicion of the origin of so remarkable a practice. Those who are acquainted with the facts of biology and the principles of therapeutics know perfectly well that the giving of a mouse to a sick child *in extremis* is no more likely to save its life than any other kind of meat diet that is tender and digestible. Such wise men would regard the giving of a mouse as a magical procedure, which indeed it is ; but this is not incompatible with the fact that originally this practice was devised on purely rational grounds, and it has become magical only because we have learned that the reasons which dictated the original use of mice as drugs are invalid.

With regard to the use of spells and incantations, in the early development of religion the oral rites came to acquire a great reputation for power ; the recitation of certain statements at the opening of the mouth of a mummy were supposed to confer life upon it. The statements of certain kings and deities were supposed to be able to confer life and to protect the lives of their subjects. It was part of a firm belief in the superhuman power of the king to do things simply by expressing a wish that they should be done. The principle is expressed very wittily by Gilbert in the opera, *The Mikado*, when the Lord High Executioner explains to the Mikado that when he ordered a certain person to be executed the execution was as good as done, and if it was as good as done it was done, and if it was done why not say so? This verbal juggling really illustrates the sort of reasoning which occurred among primitive people, and enables us the better to understand what was involved in spells and incantations as potent influences in the treatment of disease. People who had not learned that death itself was the inevitable fate of every human being, but that when it did happen it was the result of some injury to the body inflicted by some other living creature, naturally assumed that interference with the normal health of a person which was not due to any observable cause, might be produced by some creature having obtained possession of the body and requiring to be driven out in order to free the body from the element which was disturbing it. Once people got the idea that these living beings, whether we call them spirits or not matters little, occupied the body and caused these disturbances, it was perhaps not irrational to believe in the power of some verbal admonition addressed to the malicious cause of the disease to be efficacious in expelling it. Hence spells and incantations were originally simply rational systems of dealing with a particular ailment in accordance with the current theory of the etiology of the disease.

Once this idea is realized that what we call magic is simply the persistence of fallacies which were rational applications of a general theory, we will recognize that the principles underlying such primitive medicine, as recorded in the Ebers Papyrus, are not essentially different from those which inspire the treatment of disease in modern times. In both ages there were general theories of the nature of disease ; the treatment was inspired by a rational application of the knowledge in the light of this general theory. In medicine at the present time there are no doubt all sorts of fallacies both in interpreting the etiology of disease and in diagnosing it and in attempting to treat it rationally—attempts which fifty years hence may in many cases be regarded in the same way as we regard the magical practices of the past. If the growth of knowledge eliminates error, at the same time it creates magic, magic which the next generation will learn to discover and to exorcise. Hence to understand the vast accumulation of nonsensical methods of diagnosis and treatment such as those of the Ebers Papyrus, we must try to put ourselves in the position of those men thirty centuries ago who lacked the knowledge and experience our ancestors have gained in the intervening centuries, and try to sympathize with their attempts to penetrate into the elusive mysteries of constitutional disease and discover a rational means of treating it.

Leaving aside such attempts to explain Egyptian ideas, what at the moment it is more useful to do as a help towards identifying the diseases which are discussed in the Ebers Papyrus is to call attention to the actual evidence provided by the dead bodies of the ancient Egyptians of the ailments that afflicted them in the times when these ancient documents were written ; and perhaps I can best do this in the form of a personal narrative by giving a brief sketch of my own experiences in Egypt, and how I acquired a certain acquaintance with the pathological conditions which prevailed in the country at the time when the materials put together in the Ebers Papyrus were being accumulated.

A few weeks after I arrived in Egypt in 1900, my friend, the late Dr. W. H. R. Rivers, wrote to me from the camp at El Amrah, near Abydos in Upper Egypt, where Dr. Randall-MacIver and the late Mr. Anthony Wilkins were excavating a Predynastic cemetery, asking if I would be interested to see in the skulls of these people (who had died more than fifty-five centuries ago) desiccated brains so well preserved that a great many of their anatomical features were easily recognizable (Plate iii). In response to an invitation from Dr. Randall-MacIver I went to visit his camp and in the following year put on record (*Journal of Anatomy and Physiology*, July, 1902, page 375) a brief report upon the amazing phenomenon of the natural preservation of so delicate an organ as the brain.

The first Egyptian grave that I ever saw contained the skeleton of a boy in whose pelvis was a large vesical calculus (Plate iv), which Dr. Randall-MacIver generously permitted me to send to the Museum of the Royal College of Surgeons in London, where it provided the material for a very interesting pathological report by the late Professor S. G. Shattock ('A Prehistoric or Predynastic Egyptian Calculus' : *Transactions of the Pathological Society of London*, Volume 56, 1905, page 275). The discovery of a stone in the bladder several thousand years earlier than any other record of this pathological condition stimulated my interest to look for further evidence of the incidence of disease in ancient times.

A few weeks later an invitation from Professor George A. Reisner to collaborate with him in the study of the earliest human remains at that time known in Egypt, which he was bringing to light at a spot on the eastern side of the Nile (almost opposite El Amrah), on the site of the modern village of Naga-ed-Der, afforded me an exceptional opportunity for an intensive search for such information.

In this early cemetery three pathological conditions were exceptionally common : one was the incidence of arthritis ; another was a series of severe cases of mastoid disease (Plate v) ; and the third was the remarkable frequency of fracture of the ulna about two inches above the wrist, more commonly the left ulna in women, undoubtedly the result of fending with the left arm a blow from a heavy stick. The interest of this particular fracture was increased when we found on the same site in a tomb of the Second Dynasty, that is about a thousand years later, an example of the splints which were used for treating fractures of the forearm (Plate vi).

Altogether a great variety of injuries was found, which, however, I shall not attempt to enumerate.

Two of them are of particular interest. At Shellal (First Cataract), a trench outside a Roman Fort was found to contain 104 bodies of Nubians, all of whom had been executed. Most of them had been hanged, and it is interesting to note that the noose of the rope did not catch the neck as it usually does in modern hanging but the head, the bones of which were forced apart by the shock. One of these Nubians had had his head cut off with a sword.

Evidence of tubercular disease was extremely rare. Only about a dozen typical examples of tubercular caries were found in Egypt and Nubia, of which the most ancient (*circa* 2000 B.C.), and the earliest stage in the development of the disease, is shown in Plate vii.

Malignant disease was also very rare. Several cases of osteosarcoma (Plate viii) were found, three of them in the cemetery of the Fifth Dynasty at the Giza Pyramids. Evidence of only two other types of malignant disease was found—cancer of the pharynx and cancer of the rectum, both of them more than twenty centuries later than the Pyramid Age. The cancer of the throat, the former of the cases just mentioned, destroyed a large part of the base of the skull (Plate ix).

Calcareous disease of the arteries was common in all ages. The head of Rameses the Great (Plate x) shows calcified temporal arteries and also a mysterious sign painted upon the top of the scalp.

Only one case of leprosy was discovered (Plate xi) and that in a cemetery of Syrian Christians at the First Cataract.

One instance of gall-stones was found (Plate xii) in

the mummy of a Priestess of Amon (Plate xiii), who died at Thebes about 1000 B.C.

When I first visited Dr. Reisner at Naga-ed-Der he asked my advice on a curious controversy that was agitating the minds of archæologists and pathologists. A famous excavator working in the Predynastic cemeteries found injuries on many of the bones which at first sight looked like the results of gnawing, and put forward the claim that such evidence revealed the former existence of cannibalism in Egypt. A French excavator submitted similar Predynastic bones to a well-known pathologist in Lyons, who expressed the opinion that these earliest Egyptians were suffering from syphilis, a disease unknown before the Middle Ages. In *The Lancet* of August 22nd, 1908, I have published a report of the results of my inquiries into the nature of these bone-injuries that were so strangely interpreted.

Briefly the facts were that these so-called ulcers or gnawings were invariably found at the under surface of the bones as they lay in the ground, and in several cases burrows leading through the soil could be traced to the damaged patches. On examining the edges of the so-called ulcers with a lens, it was shown that the gnawing was due neither to human teeth nor to the spirochæte, but to small necrophilous beetles which had produced these injuries long after the burial of the bodies. As a matter of fact, after examining the remains of something like thirty-thousand bodies of ancient Egyptians and Nubians, representing every period in the history of the last sixty centuries, and from every part of the country, it can be stated quite confidently that no trace whatever even suggesting syphilitic injuries to bones or teeth was revealed in Egypt before modern times. Nor was any case of true rickets found in a human skeleton, although in some domestic animals, in particular some of the sacred monkeys kept in a temple of Thebes, distortions suggestive of rickets were found.

Both in Nubia and Egypt the ordinary form of dental caries was exceedingly rare in Predynastic and Protodynastic times, and among the poorer classes it never became at all common until modern times. However, as these people ate coarse food mixed with a considerable amount of sand the teeth became rapidly worn down, and very often the pulp-cavities were exposed. In the fertile soil of the exposed dental pulp, septic infection found a much readier means of attack than the hard resisting enamel and dentine of the tooth itself afforded ; hence it is common to find alveolar abscesses without dental caries (Plate xiv). Most of the dental diseases of the archaic Egyptians and the poorer classes of the ancient Nubians is to be explained in this way.

Dental caries, although extremely rare before the Pyramid Age, became common as soon as people learned luxury. In the cemetery of the time of the ancient Empire excavated by the Hearst Expedition at the Giza Pyramids, more than five hundred skeletons of aristocrats of the time of the pyramid-builders (*circa* 2800 B.C.) were brought to light, and in these bodies it was found that tartar-formation, dental caries, and alveolar abscesses were at least as common as they are in modern Europe to-day. At every subsequent period of Egyptian history one finds the same thing—the wide prevalence of every form of dental disease among the wealthy people who indulge in a luxurious diet, and the relative immunity from such ailments among the poorer people who lived mainly on a coarse uncooked vegetable diet. There is in no case the slightest suggestion that any operative measures were adopted in order to cope with dental trouble, and in spite of frequent statements to the contrary, tooth-stopping was never practised in ancient Egypt. Even the mummy of Amenophis III, often called The Magnificent, who reigned at a time when Egyptian power and luxury had attained their fullest expression, revealed no trace of any attempt to deal with the extreme condition of caries and alveolar inflammation found in his jaws.

The most remarkable controversy that developed out of the study of the Royal mummies is of special interest and even now, nearly twenty years after the event, is not yet settled. It was concerned with the heretic king, Akhenaton. The late Mr. Theodore Davis, who financed the excavations in the Valley of the Tombs of the Kings near Thebes from 1903 to 1912 often stated that his chief ambition was to discover the tomb of the famous Queen Tiy, the wife of the Pharaoh Amenophis III of the Eighteenth Dynasty.

In 1907 the announcement was made (by Professor

Sayce) in a letter to *The Times* that Mr. Davis had found the tomb of the famous Queen. I knew nothing more about this matter until about three months later, when, in July 1907, the Inspector of Antiquities in Upper Egypt, Mr. Arthur Weigall, sent to me in Cairo a box containing a skeleton which he said was all that was left of the famous Queen. On opening this box to my intense surprise I found not the bones of an old lady but those of a young man and I at once telegraphed to Luxor to Mr. Weigall to say that he had sent the wrong skeleton, for the bones were those of a young man. In reply to this I received the somewhat cryptic reply in one word, 'Splendid.' I discovered afterwards that throughout the course of the excavation Mr. Weigall had maintained that the tomb was not that of the famous Queen, but her son's, the heretic king, Akhenaton's. The archæological evidence seemed to leave no room for doubt that the bones were actually those of the heretic king, but a difficulty now arose from the consideration that the anatomical evidence seemed to point to an age of about twenty-three (or at most thirty, if the process of development had been exceptionally delayed), whereas the historical evidence suggested that Akhenaton was at least thirty, and in all probability thirty-six years of age.

In considering this difficult problem I naturally turned to consider those pathological conditions which might cause the delay in the union of the epiphyses. Of these the most likely seemed to be the syndrome described by Froehlich in 1901 which is now known as dystrophia adiposo-genitalis. In this condition the bones at thirty-six years of age may still persist in a condition which in the normal individual they reach at twenty-two or twenty-three. Hence this suggested one possibility of bringing the anatomical evidence into harmony with the historical data. In support of this suggestion there is the very peculiar anatomical features of Akhenaton when alive, which have been made familiar to us by a large series of contemporary portraits. These pictures reveal features found in Froehlich's syndrome and afford valuable support of the suggestion that this was the real cause for the delay in the fusion of the epiphyses. In addition to this, the skull (Plate xv)—both the brain case and face —revealed certain important peculiarities. There is a slight degree of hydrocephalus, such as is often associated with the development of Froehlich's syndrome, and also the overgrowth of the mandible that results from interference with the pituitary.

The full solution of this problem cannot be made until the bones are submitted to a much fuller investigation than I was permitted to make in 1907, but when this has been accomplished the solution of a comparatively simple anatomical problem will throw a decisive light upon one of the most critical events in the whole history of civilization ; one which was charged with the fate of all the ruling nations of the world at that time and which left its impress upon the history of the world at large.

It is only right to say that this diagnosis has been suggested only after a very careful consideration of all the relevant facts, historical and anatomical, and a sifting of all the possibilities of interpretation. In the volume (*The Royal Mummies*) which I contributed to the General Catalogue of the Cairo Museum in 1912, I have made a full statement of all the evidence that was then available concerning the remains of Akhenaton's skeleton and in 1923 I discussed its significance in my little book, *Tutankhamen*. The slight hydrocephalus (Plate xv), the indication of an early overgrowth of the jaw such as occurs in acromegaly, and the gradual assumption of a feminine contour of figure, with a delayed union of the epiphyses, suggest the possibility that the solution of the problem of Akhenaton may be provided by the diagnosis of dystrophia adiposo-genitalis.

This diagnosis, however, does not go unchallenged, and certain criticisms were raised when (on January 18th, 1928) I discussed this interesting problem in an address to the medical students at Westminster Hospital (Guthrie Society), which was published in their journal, *Broadway* (Spring 1928, page 25).

It was argued that Akhenaton could not have been the father of three daughters whom he is so often depicted as fondling with paternal pride, if he had been afflicted with the sterility that usually goes with adiposo-genital dystrophy. A possible explanation of this difficulty may be found in the fact that the onset of the dystrophy may not have occurred until after the birth of his daughters. Of the life-history of no king of Egypt have we so complete a record as of Akhenaton's. The sculptors of his time made a series of portrait statues and bas-reliefs which depict him at various stages of his career. Fortunately, also, art at this period had become freed from the shackles of convention so that the actual appearance of Akhenaton is revealed to us naturally and realistically at different ages. If we accept them as true representations of his personal appearance we can assert that he was not abnormal in his 'teens,' and that the dystrophy must have gradually developed after he was twenty. If this is the true history there is no reason why he might not between the ages of fifteen to twenty have been the father of these children whom he obviously treated as his offspring.

I am not competent to express an authoritative opinion on the symptoms and results of this dystrophy. Some years ago, however, before venturing to suggest it as the only possible explanation I could discover to eliminate the apparent conflict between the anatomical and the historical evidence, I consulted the full report on the history and manifestations of dystrophia adiposo-genitalis, written by Dr. Harvey G. Beck in Professor Llewellyn F. Barker's *Endocrinology and Metabolism* (Volume I, page 859, New York, 1922). It seems to me that the actual cases reported by Dr. Beck afford a possible explanation of all we know of Akhenaton's symptoms, and also an answer to the objections that have been raised against the suggested diagnosis of adiposo-genital dystrophy as the solution of the enigma his case presents. Sterility is not an invariable result of this dystrophy, in certain victims of which either the excessive development of fat or the genital disability may be present without the other.

In these notes I have attempted to summarize what little we know of the incidence of disease in ancient Egypt, not merely such complaints as arthritis and mastoid disease which are mentioned in the Ebers Papyrus, but also of other ailments that have not been recognized in the writings. It is now coming to be recognized that studies in Egyptian philology alone are not likely to solve the difficulties of interpretation of the medical papyri. The survival in Egypt and elsewhere of ancient archaic terms and ancient remedies is pointing the way to the understanding of much that otherwise would be obscure in the Egyptian texts. As I have already stated the comparative study of folk-lore and herbals, the investigation of mediæval leechdom and pharmacopœias, is providing information for the identification of diseases and drugs and a welcome illumination of the principles underlying the ancient physician's methods of practice.

Hence Dr. Bryan's book, even if it does no more than direct attention to the general nature of the contents of the Egyptian medical documents, will serve the useful purpose of appealing to students of folk-lore and archæology, of herbals and theology, to be alert for clues which may solve problems of exceptional interest that appeal to the deepest desires of every human being to safeguard health and life itself.

Since the foregoing paragraphs have been printed Professor James Henry Breasted's sumptuous monograph on the Edwin Smith Surgical Papyrus—the result of ten years' intensive investigation—has been published by the University of Chicago Press. Hence it is no longer correct to say that no Ancient Egyptian treatise on Medicine has been translated into English. Moreover Professor Breasted's work is the most ambitious attempt that has ever been made to interpret an ancient medical treatise, for he has summoned to his aid all the resources of Egyptian philology and used his superb scholarship and insight to discover the subtle meaning underlying the cryptic phraseology. He has provided all the material on the Egyptian side so that the way is now ready to institute comparisons with Hebrew and Greek literature and, using the technique of Professor Yahouda's method, bring illumination to the writings of these three ancient peoples, to whom in different ways our own civilization is so deeply indebted.

The issue of Professor Breasted's treatise does not minimize the need for such works of popularization as Dr. Bryan's. On the contrary the increased interest the former will provoke should extend the demand for such guide-books as the latter.

G. Elliot Smith.

University College,
London.
August, 1930

AUTHOR'S FOREWORD

Little more than fifty years ago there came into the possession of a German Egyptologist a roll of papyrus that was destined to prove the oldest book the world possesses. It could not have fallen into worthier hands, for within three years there issued in two beautiful volumes not only a facsimile of the whole papyrus but, as well, a German translation and a Hieroglypho-Latin glossary : the whole work constituting a monument to German scholarship that commands the admiration of all time.

And yet, after a lapse of more than half a century, the English-speaking student seeks in vain an English translation of this most ancient of books !

* * *

It is incredible. A country so intimately connected with Egypt, whose most treasured possessions reflect the culture and the glory of that ancient land, and which has produced so many eminent men skilled in the lore and learning of Egypt cannot afford to ignore for ever this document that has come to us from out the very womb of time. It is not that the Papyrus is inaccessible. As fresh and as perfect as when it was penned some four thousand years ago it reposes to-day in the library of the University of Leipzig, while every library of note throughout the civilized world boasts at least one of those beautiful facsimile editions which we owe to the discoverer's unquenchable energy. And it is not that its value has decreased with the years, for it still remains the most ancient complete book in the world. Can it be that the task is too great?

* * *

To be sure the preparation of a complete English edition will be no easy task. One of our greatest Egyptologists, F. L. Griffith, writing in 1893, has put on record his opinion of the sort of man who, only, could cope *successfully* with it. In the first place he must be a Physician: for a knowledge of Anatomy, Physiology, and Nosology, in a *sine qua non*. Then he must be familiar with the Egyptian language and in sympathy with the ideas and methods of these ancient peoples; he must have a knowledge of the substances likely to be available and used as medicinal compounds; he must be conversant not only with Savage and Primitive Medicine but with Classical and Mediæval Practice as well, since they were so interwoven. Lastly, he must bring to bear on the work a knowledge of modern Egyptian diseases and their native treatment.

Then, having so admirably arrayed the qualifications needed for the task, Griffith bluntly proceeded to declare that no one person possessed them all.

* * *

But even were that true—and it probably was, and is, true—that constitutes no warrant for shirking the responsibility. Though there be no one person to combine in himself all the qualifications that would go to a perfect interpretation into English of the letter and the spirit of the Papyrus Ebers, it is not very difficult to imagine that the scientific world could produce three or four men who, working in concert, could encompass the task. It is unfortunate that Griffith himself did not see his way clear to amplify the partial translations that he has published on occasions ; it is more than unfortunate, it is a distinct loss—especially when we observe that same scholar's translations of those fragments of medical papyri in the British Museum, dating back a thousand years earlier than the Papyrus Ebers.

But he has not done it, neither he nor those others whose life-long studies and researches should have fitted them for the task. Until they do so, the English-speaking student is offered this little volume, a rendition into English of German and other translations of the Egyptian original.

* * *

One word more. Most Ancient of *Books* is the claim made for the Papyrus Ebers ; not, be it noted, Most Ancient of *Papyri*. Not (by more than two thousand years) can it claim the latter distinction. Indeed, scattered about the museums and libraries of Europe there are in point of fact a score or more of papyri, all of them centuries older than the Papyrus Ebers. But these papyri are not *books*, any more than a leaf or several leaves torn from a modern volume constitute the volume itself. For the most part they are scraps of papyrus, torn and bedraggled and much the worse for wear by their passage through the ages, and only partly legible. The papyrus discovered by Ebers, however, complete to the most minute detail, and legible from first to last, is a book, a real book, and nothing but a book, and, as clearly on this ground as on the score of age, justifies the claim made for it to be the Most Ancient Book in the World.

CYRIL BRYAN.

THE PAPYRUS EBERS

Chapter I

AGE OF THE PAPYRUS

It was in the winter of 1872 that the German Egyptologist, Georg Ebers, came into possession of the papyrus which according to the usual custom bears his name. Whilst excavating in the vicinity of Thebes he was one day approached by a wealthy Egyptian, who, so he discovered, had made the journey from Luxor expressly to see him. When however the Egyptian produced nothing more exciting than a practically worthless papyrus and a modern statue of Osiris, Ebers suspicions were aroused and he diplomatically informed his visitor that he was prepared to pay handsomely for anything of value that was being held back. The Egyptian thereupon disappeared.

The next day he reappeared and handed to Ebers a metal case. Inside, wrapped in old mummy-cloths, was a papyrus the sight of which must have taken the Egyptologist's breath away. The huge roll was in a perfect state of preservation ; the writing, both red and black, stood out as clear and vivid as if but written the previous day ; and a calendar on the back of the first page indicated a date at the very latest a thousand years before Christ ! But Ebers' joy was to be tempered with a little uncertainty. The Egyptian had some idea of the value of his property and fixed the price accordingly. It was beyond Ebers, and for a time the fate of the precious manuscript trembled in the balance. However, the timely appearance of a wealthy compatriot, Herr Gunther, disposed of the financial difficulty ; and in a few days Ebers was returning hot-foot to Germany to deposit his treasure in the Library of the University of Leipzig. As already stated, in less than three years he had not only translated it into German but had given it to the world in facsimile in two wonderful volumes ; while his friend and companion, Stern, had enriched the work beyond measure by appending a Hieroglypho-Latin glossary.

The age of the Papyrus was for Ebers the first consideration. From the beginning the calendar on the reverse of the front page had exercised him far more than the perfect preservation or the beauty of the document. But it was not to give up its secret without a struggle, and its interpretation exercised all the ingenuity of its finder. It was the irony of fate that he should have missed by a few years the man who could have made plain most of the puzzle—who could in all probability have opened a new and intensely interesting chapter of Egyptian history—this was the native who only fourteen years previously had discovered the Papyrus between the legs of a mummy in a tomb at El Assassif, near Thebes . . . and then died ! However, by the time the publisher was ready with his facsimile edition in 1875, Ebers was able to declare 'with a probability bordering on certainty,' that his Papyrus dated from the years 1553-1550 B.C. Challenged at first in various quarters, the date fixed by Ebers has since been definitely confirmed by such authorities as Ehrmann of Berlin, and Griffith of Oxford, both of whom have identified the King in whose reign it was transcribed as Amen-Hotep I, a Pharaoh of the Eighteenth Dynasty, who reigned in Egypt exactly two hundred years before the now familiar Tut-Ankh-Amen came to the throne.

But Ebers was not content with merely fixing the date : he claimed that his Papyrus was nothing less than one of the 'Hermetic Books' of the Ancient Egyptians, in fact the only one then known.

Clement of Alexandria writing in A.D. 200, and again Iamblichus in A.D. 363, recorded that the Egyptian priests possessed forty-two books in which was contained the sum of Human Knowledge. These books were called by the Greeks the 'Hermetic Books,' because their authorship was ascribed to the god Hermes : Hermes being the Greek name for the god who in the Egyptian Pantheon was known as Thoth, God of the Healing Art. But it was not as a god that Thoth had gathered the sum of Human Knowledge into these so-called Hermetic Books ; on the contrary it was because he had as an ordinary (or extraordinary!) mortal done this great service that he was acclaimed a god by a grateful people and raised to the Pantheon as the God of the Healing Art. Exactly who he was in his mortal state is not clear. He is identified by various authorities with Athothis, 3,400 B.C., who besides being a mighty king was learned in all the arts and sciences ; and with Imhotep, who also excelled in every branch of learning, especially in the mysteries of the healing art. Both these personages were deified because of their excellent qualities, and it is quite within the realm of possibility that both were one and the same person. The point, however, does not concern us here.

Of these forty-two books, Clement tells us, thirty-six dealt with Philosophy and General Knowledge, whilst the last six were devoted to the Healing Art under the following heads :

Book 37. Anatomy.
" 38. Diseases.
" 39. Surgery.
" 40. Remedies.
" 41. Diseases of the Eye.
" 42. Diseases of Women.

The Book of Remedies, Book 40, is the document Ebers believed he had re-discovered. But the claim was not received without challenge. Joachim definitely rejected the claim on the ground that the Papyrus was not an 'original,' but merely a Medical Compendium, i.e., a collection of remedies gathered from various sources. Why the fact that it was not an 'original' precludes it from being one of the Hermetic Books mentioned by Clement of Alexandria is hard to understand. Ebers never for a moment claimed that it was an 'original' in the strict sense, and he was the first to draw attention to various entries that proved beyond doubt that the Scribe had copied from earlier, or at least from other writings. For example, on Plates 18,

89 and 90, he showed us, interpolated in the text, the Hieratic characters, Qem Sen, meaning 'found destroyed,' the reference in each instance being to a remedy which the Scribe was on that account unable to give in its entirety. Again, it would hardly be seriously suggested that the Hermetic Books possessed by the Egyptian Priests at the time when Clement wrote, two hundred years after Christ, were the selfsame unaltered originals that were written by Imhotep (or Athothis, or whoever it was who wrote them) three thousand years previously! That they were added to and amended and re-written during the course of thirty centuries goes without saying, and the claim made by Ebers has yet to be refuted on stronger ground than this.

However, the value of the Papyrus Ebers does not rest on its claim to be the sole survivor of the Hermetic Books, and Joachim hastened to qualify his rejection of that claim by the assertion that it did not lessen by one iota the immense value of the document. Of that he left no doubt: witness his summing up of the Papyrus:

> 'It surpasses in importance all other medical papyri in the richness of its contents and its completeness and perfection. It is the largest, the most beautifully written, and the best preserved of all the medical papyri.'

Chapter II

DESCRIPTION OF THE PAPYRUS

The Papyrus as Ebers first saw it was in one long roll, twelve inches in width and sixty-eight feet in length. Throughout its whole length it was divided into what may be called ' pages,' each of equal size and averaging twenty lines apiece. Each page was numbered at its head and a glance at the last page gave the idea that there were 110 such pages in the manuscript. But a closer inspection page by page revealed a strange irregularity. Page 27 was found to be followed by page 30 without any break in the continuity of the text ; there was no page 28 nor page 29 ! The reason for the omission of these numbers in the paging is not apparent. While Joachim dismisses it as a mere oversight, Griffith declares it to be intentional on the part of the Scribe who wished the Papyrus to finish on the number 110, a figure considered to be a ' perfect number ' by the ancient Egyptians.

While Ebers and the other Egyptologists were wrestling with its age and deciphering its contents, the Papyrus was undergoing a drastic metamorphosis and the Scribe who laboriously inscribed its sixty-eight feet of length would be considerably startled could he see the result of his labours as it reposes to-day in its up-to-date dress in the University Library of Leipzig. It is no longer a roll of Papyrus. Its pages have been carefully cut and bound in modern form, its preservation thus insured to the utmost, and its accessibility to students amplified a thousandfold.

He would be dull of soul indeed who could remain unmoved even by the mere description of this Most Ancient of Books. But one need not content oneself with the mere description : its wonders and its beauty are realistically portrayed in the facsimile edition of Ebers to be viewed in the manuscript room of the British Museum.

As one turns over the Plates that go to make up these two volumes, the mind is bewildered by the multitude of thoughts and impressions which are called up. Above all is the feeling of awe, or reverent awe, for the Scribe whose graceful, easy writing, without fault or flaw holds us enthralled. From beginning to end of the Papyrus not a line, not a word, not even a letter, is missing ; so that after a lapse of thirty-four centuries his infinite patience and his artistry are there for us to admire in their entirety.

The first thing that catches the eye on examining the Papyrus is the touch of colour given to it by reason of the 'Rubrics,' the red capitals with which the beginning of each chapter and paragraph is enriched. There was a time when we were accustomed to think that this fashion of Rubrics grew, like many other things, out of the Middle Ages, but a glance at almost any of the ancient Egyptian papyri quickly dispels that idea. Throughout the manuscript the headings of the different chapters, the names of the diseases, the directions for treatment, and in many cases the weights and dosages of the drugs are written in a vivid red which holds its colour to-day every whit as fast as does the black in the text.

An understanding of the Papyrus Ebers, or of any Egyptian papyrus, involves an excursion into the domain of Philology. A most interesting excursion it is.

The Papyrus Ebers is of course written in the Hieratic, which is a cursive script evolved in course of time from the Hieroglyphics that excite our curiosity on the ancient Egyptian monuments. These Hieroglyphics were eminently suited for chiselling out of stone, but when it came to writing them down on paper, or rather papyri, it was a vastly different matter. To trace minutely on to papyrus the quaint birds and beasts and other objects which went to make up the Hieroglyphic vocabulary, entailed not only great patience, it must have involved an appalling amount of time. Our imagination can easily and with practical certainty bridge over the gap between Hieroglyphics and Hieratic. At first the fine points of the Hieroglyphics, unconsciously perhaps, were slurred over ; and this first step being taken the rest was only a matter of time. The slurring became conscious, was recognized as inevitable, and finally the Scribes found themselves in possession of a flowing cursive style of writing that we know to-day as Hieratic.

But this evolution did not stop at the Hieratic stage, which was in fact the script of the Priests, or learned class. The final stage was reached apparently about the Eighth Century B.C., when we find the common people in possession of a folk-script called Demotic, which from its presence on the famous Rosetta Stone was destined to play a prominent part in the unravelling of the literature of ancient Egypt. Prior to the discovery of the Rosetta Stone in 1799, or it should be said to its unravelling in 1822, ancient Egyptian literature was practically a closed book to us. The Rosetta Stone, however, supplied the key, for inscribed on it were Hieroglyphic characters with both their Demotic and Greek equivalents, and it only awaited the coming of the English physicist and physician, Thomas Young, and of the great French Egyptologist, Champollion, and others, to reveal to us an intimate knowledge of that other world which up till then had meant little more to us than Pyramids, Sphinxes, and Tombs.

To return to our Papyrus. Since the Hieratic was not inscribed on the Rosetta Stone it was necessary in the first place to translate the Hieratic of the Papyrus into Hieroglyphics. Thence by means of the Demotic and the Greek its meaning was worked out of the inky darkness in which it had remained for thousands of years. On the Plates shown in this volume this rendering of the Hieratic into Hieroglyphics of men, birds, and beasts, can be plainly traced in the Hieratic script (written it will be noted from right to left) and the study will prove an education in itself, well repaying the time spent on it.

Chapter III

CONTENTS OF THE PAPYRUS

For the most part the Papyrus Ebers is devoted to the medicinal treatment of diseases, surgical interference being recommended in only about a score of cases. The pathological conditions range from the Sting of a Wasp to the Bite of a Crocodile, from a trivial ache to the most loathsome disease. The Anatomy, Physiology and Pathology of the Heart and Circulatory System are dealt with in a special chapter ; morbid conditions of the Alimentary and Urinary tracts are gone into very thoroughly ; Obstetrics and Gynæcology have no complaint on the score of neglect ; the Skin, the Teeth, the Ears, and especially the Eyes, receive due attention.

In addition quite an extensive amount of space is given to Cosmetics. We find remedies to drive out wrinkles and to make the face smooth, to remove moles and to beautify the body, to alter the colour of the skin and to dye the hair and eyebrows, to make the hair grow, to correct 'squint.' Then in all sorts of unexpected places we pick up handy hints in the shape of recipes to kill scorpions and lizards, to stop the pigeon-hawk stealing, to keep rats out of the granary, to prevent the serpent creeping out of his hole, to charm away fleas, lice, and mice, to soothe a crying baby, to prognosticate the fate of a new-born child, to distinguish spoiled milk, to sweeten the breath—these and numerous others being rounded off by a remedy for sweaty feet !

The following summary of the pathological conditions described or dealt with in the Papyrus will afford a better idea as to its scope, an attempt having been made to group them in some sort of order. To Joachim even more than to Ebers are we indebted for the fact that it is possible to prepare such a list. A scholar, an Egyptologist, and a physician, he bent his whole mind to the task of giving to the world in a modern tongue, not only a word-for-word translation of the precious document but of elucidating many passages which without such elucidation would be to us so much gibberish ; and it was only after diligent study and research extending over years that he was enabled to diagnose the actual complaints from the descriptions often so cryptically supplied by the Scribe :

Headache
Migraine
Giddiness
Constipation
Diarrhœa
Indigestion
Colic
Dysentery
Melæna
Piles

Inflammations of the Anus
Tumours and Inflammations of the Abdomen
Tapeworms
Roundworms
Guinea-worm
Hookworm
Polyuria
Frequency of Micturition
Accumulation and Obstruction of Urine
Cystitis
Enlarged Prostate
Stricture
Stone
Cardiac pain and weakness
Palpitation
Disorderly Action of the Heart
Atheroma
Debility
Diseases of the Liver
Glandular swellings
Tumours, innocent and malignant
Fat Tumours
Skin Tumours
Tumours of Nerves and Vessels
Baldness
Alopecia
Scurf
Eczema
Impetigo
Scabies
Stings of Wasps and Tarantulæ

Bite of a Crocodile
Burns of the First, Second, Third, Fourth, and Fifth Day
Wounds
Abscesses
Gangrene
Pustules and Suppurations
Menstrual irregularities
Amenorrhœa
Leucorrhœa
Aids to Delivery, Abortion, and Lactation
Diseases of the Breasts
Falling of the Womb
Ulcers and Diseases of the Female genitalia
Teeth irregularities
Gumboils and Abscesses
Coryza
Catarrh
Diseases of the Tongue
Deafness
Discharges from, and Ulcerations of, the Ear
Eye-diseases, of which Ebers has described
Blindness
Blepharitis
Cancer
Chemosis
Chalazion
Cataract
Ectropion
Entropion
Granulations

Hæmorrhage
Hydrophthalmus
Inflammations
Iritis
Leucoma
Ophthalmoplegia
Pinguecula
Pterygium
Staphyloma
Trichiasis

Chapter IV

THE PHARMACOPŒIA OF ANCIENT EGYPT

Altogether 811 prescriptions are set forth in the Papyrus, and they take the form of salves, plasters, and poultices ; snuffs, inhalations, and gargles ; draughts, confections, and pills ; fumigations, suppositories, and enemata.

A few of the prescriptions are extremely simple, only one substance being directed to be taken, or applied as a plaster or poultice, or rubbed in. The majority, however, are more complex and run from half a dozen to a dozen or more drugs ; while one on Plate 83 consists of thirty-seven ingredients. Many of the preparations, even if we cannot credit them with any therapeutic effect, appear at least to be harmless ; other remedies such as the application of Raw Meat to a Black Eye present a more up-to-date touch ; but there are over many which can only be described as curious in the highest degree.

A glance through the pharmacopœia on which the Papyrus Ebers is based is not to be undertaken lightly. To be sure we encounter there a number of drugs that figure in our pharmacopœia to-day, but they are dwarfed by the weird and wonderful substances that the Scribe gravely transcribes. It is here that we first make acquaintance with that God-given drug, Castor Oil, which besides finding itself in a hundred prescriptions has the honour of a special mention in the body of the book :

MEMORANDUM ON THE USE OF THE CASTOR OIL TREE (AS FOUND IN THE ANCIENT WRITINGS OF THE WISE MEN)

When a Person rubs its Stalk in Water and applies it to a Head which is Diseased, he will immediately become as if he had never been ill.

When a Person who suffers from Constipation chews a little of its Berry along with Beer, then the Disease will be driven out of the Sick One's body.

Also, a Woman's Hair will increase in growth by using the Berries. She crushes them, makes them into one, puts them in Oil, and anoints her Head therewith.

Furthermore, the Oil from its Berries is pressed out as an Ointment for the use of any Person who has the uha-abscess-with-stinking-matter. Lo, the Evil will fly as though he had suffered nothing ! For Ten Days he anoints himself afresh daily in the morning in order to drive the abscess away.

But extolled though it was these ancient physicians were not satisfied with Castor Oil alone, and in their search for the wherewithal to fight the disease which afflicted the land they reached as high as the heavens, actually prescribing Excrement-of-the-Gods ; and as low as—well, as low as the following pages will reveal. They laid heavy hands on the animal world, on the mineral world, on the plant world, and not least on the World of Fancy ; and having got a substance which they imagined possessed the slightest therapeutic virtue they prescribed it internally and externally, raw and cooked, ripe and unripe ; in some cases over-ripe and actually rotting. They would take a plant or a tree and strip it of its blossoms and its flowers, its fruit and its nuts, its leaves and its bark, its thorns if it had any, its stem, its root, and the bark of its root, its sap, its resin, and its fat. Even then they were not finished with it ; they collected any splinters of it that survived and used them (will it be believed ?) as a poultice for their *nerves* ! And when the plant was capable of no further dismemberment they directed that the particular one used should come from the North or from the South as their fancy moved them, from Upper or from Lower Egypt, from the Hills or from the Delta, from the Fields or from the Meadows or from the Marshes. Their ingenuity not yet exhausted, they turned their attention to the administration of the remedies, exhibiting again a versatility in every way comparable to their pharmaceutical efforts. Thus, we read of the mother who was instructed to spit the remedy into the child's mouth, of the woman who was ordered to take her medicine while she sat cross-legged, and of that other lady who, after chanting the Magic Formula, was told to have coitus before swallowing the medicament.

A final reference must be made to the vehicles by which it was sought to make the nauseous mixtures and objectionable messes which passed for poultices less nauseous and less objectionable. These vehicles, Beer, Milk, and Water, were employed with well balanced impartiality ; they were often to be found in the same concoction ; they appear in all sorts of forms, recognizable and unrecognizable. Thus Beer, a favourite vehicle, was prescribed as Plain Beer, Sweet Beer, Bitter Beer, Cold Beer, Warmed Beer, Flat Beer, Yeast-of-Beer, Froth-of-Beer, Beer-which-has-been-Brewed-from-many-Ingredients ; while in a bright moment they bethought themselves of Swill-of-Beer. Milk also afforded them some scope ; it appears as Fresh Milk, Sour Milk, Spoiled Milk, Cooked Milk, Ass's Milk, Cow's Milk, Man's Milk, Milk-of-a-Woman, Milk-of-a-Woman-who-has-borne-a-Son, Milk-of-the-Sycamore, and Milk-juice. As for Water, we find Plain Water, Well Water, Spring Water, Salt Water, Mineral Water, Cake Water, Linseed Water, Natron Water, Water-from-the-Bird-Pond, Water-from-the-Rain-of-the-Heavens, and—Water-in-which-the-Phallus-has-been-Washed !

CHAPTER V

MINERAL REMEDIES

To attempt anything more than roughly to subdivide the 'drugs' that go to the making of this pharmacopœia would be as unnecessary as it would be unprofitable. It is sufficient to place them under three main headings, Mineral, Plant, and Animal. As regards the first-named, with which this chapter deals, and under which heading are grouped various other substances which are even more foreign to the Plant and Animal worlds—few of them are prescribed in their crude or native state. Antimony, Calamine, Granite, Ink, Indigo, and Sulphur almost exhaust the list. Outside of these the source of origin of the drugs is strictly laid down, or various preparations made from the parent drug are prescribed. Thus, the Iron must be Iron-from-Apollonopolis-parva ; the Leather must be Leather-from-the-Sandal-maker ; the Soot must be Soot-from-the-bet'a-pot ; the Soda must be Soda-from-Upper-Egypt. But it were better to set them down in some sort of order, alphabetical preferably.

Alabaster
Meal-of-Alabaster
Dust-of-Alabaster

Antimony

An-old-Book-cooked-in-Oil

Bread
Bread-crumbs
Bread-dough
Bread-meal
Fragrant Bread
Fermenting Bread
Bread-of-the-Zizyphus-Lotus

Cake
A-portion-of-Cake
Cake-meal
Cake-water

Calamine

Clay-from-the-Gate
Clay-from-a-Statue
Clay-from-the-Wall
Mason's Clay

Collyrium

Copper
Copper-coal
Copper-rust
Copper-shavings
Copper-vitriol

Copper-verdigris

Dough

The-Film-of-Dampness-which-is-Found-on-the-Wood-of-Ships

Granite

Gum-water
Drops-of-Gum

Hæmatite
Honey
Fresh Honey
Wild Honey
Honeycomb

Indigo

Iron-from-Apollonopolis-parva

Lapis lazuli
Real Lapis lazuli

Lead
Lead-vitriol
Fresh Lead-earth

Leather-from-the-Sandal-maker

Myrrh
Dried Myrrh
Sweet Myrrh
Oil-of-Myrrh

Natron
Red Natron
Refined Natron
Natron-water
Meal-of-Natron

Oil
Castor Oil
Olive Oil
White Oil
Oil-of-Two-Days
Oil-of-the-Earth (Petroleum)
Oil-from-the-Top-of-the-des-jar
Pieces-of-dried Oil

Opal-resin

Salt
Fresh Salt
Mineral Salt
Sea-salt
Salt-from-the-North

Saltpetre
Saltpetre-from-the-South
Saltpetre-from-Upper-Egypt

Scrapings-from-a-Statue
Dust-of-a-Statue

Soot-from-the-bet'a-pot

Stone-from-the-Shore
Stone-from-the-Meeting-of-the-Waters
Stone-from-the-Parting-of-the-Waters
Stone-from-Memphis
Knife-stone
Black Knife-stone
Trash-from-the-Knife-Stone

Sulphur

Verdigris
Copper-verdigris

Wax
Ibis-of-Wax

Writing-fluid

Yeast
Yeast-of-Wine
Yeast-of-Beer
Yeast-of-Sweet-Beer
Yeast-of-Bitter-Beer
Yeast-of-Beer-that-is-Fermenting
Yeast-of-Beer-that-has-Fermented

Yeast-of-Beer-that-has-been-whipped-up
Yeast-of-the-Opium-drink

Included in the above list is the substance Hæmatite and the positive identification of this "drug" is interesting and illustrative of the difficulties that beset the original translators of the Egyptian Papyri. The Egyptian word for this is *d'd'* (or *didi*) and it was originally translated as the Mandrake (or love-apple) on account of its resemblance to the Hebrew word *dudaim* in the Old Testament. For many years this was accepted without question until in the *Evolution of the Dragon* (1919) Professor G. Elliot Smith drew public attention to the error. Gauthier's researches, he pointed out, had led him to the conclusion that *didi* was nothing else but red clay, while Griffith had gone further and properly identified the substance as red ochre or hæmatite. In 1927 Dawson in the Journal of the Royal Asiatic Society gave a comprehensive summary of the occurrence of and the use to which *didi* was put in most of the Egyptian Papyri. He appears to have clinched the matter for good and all, consequently no mention of the Mandrake will be found in these pages, the *alraunen* of the German translations being interpreted as Hæmatite.

Chapter VI

PLANT REMEDIES

The foregoing by no means constitute a full list of the Mineral substances employed in the pharmacopœia, for there are many others whose identity is completely hidden from us under the guise of meaningless words which are beyond the comprehension of the many Egyptologists who have from time to time wrestled with the Papyrus. This is unfortunate to the point of annoyance at times, and it applies equally to those substances which were drawn from the Plant world. However, of the recognizable Plants, and of their preparations, there is a not inconsiderable showing as the following list will reveal.

Acanthus-tree
Dough-of-Acanthus
Fruit-of-Acanthus
Nuts-of-Acanthus
Resin-of-Acanthus
Thorns-of-Acanthus

Aloes
Grain-of-Aloes

Resin-of-Aloes
Wood-of-Aloes

Arabian-wood Powder

Balsam
Real Balsam

Barley-plant

Beans
Dried Beans

Caraway
Caraway-seeds

Cedar-tree
Fat-of-the-Cedar-tree
Splinters-of-the-Cedar-tree
Tops-of-the-Cedar-tree

Rotted Cereals

Chopped-up Chaff

Coriander
Coriander-berries

Corn
Red Corn

Crocus
Crocus-from-the-South
Crocus-from-the-Hills
Crocus-from-the-Delta

Cucumber
Flowers-of-the-Cucumber

Cyperus-from-the-North
Cyperus-from-the-Fields
Cyperus-from-the-Meadow
Cyperus-from-the-Marshes
Knots-of-the-Cyperus
Thorns-of-the-Cyperus
Cyperus-grass

Dates
Fresh Dates
Green Dates
Wild Dates
Date-meal
Date-juice
Juice-of-the-Wild-Date
Dates-of-the-Male-Palm
Dates-of-the-Dompalm
Refuse-of-Dates

Ebonywood
Shavings-of-Ebonywood

Edelkraut

Elderberry

Fennel

Figs

Flax-plant
Stem-of-the-Flax-plant
Refuse-of-Flax-plant

Garlic

Grapes

Gruel
Freshly-cooked Gruel

Herbs-of-the-Field

Juniper-berries

Lettuce
Wild Lettuce

Linseed
Linseed-water

Mint-of-the-Mountains

Splinters-of-the-Mulberry-tree

Nasturtium

Onions
Fresh Onions
Green Onions
Onions-from-the-Oasis
Onion-meal
Inner-of-Onions
Sap-of-Fresh-Onions

Palm-tree
Palm-juice
Palm-fibres
Fruit-of-the-Male-Palm
Fruit-of-the-Dompalm

Papyrus-plant

Blossoms-of-the-Peppermint

Bark-of-the-Pomegranate
Bark-of-the-Pomegranate-tree-soaked-in-Beer

Poppy-plant
Poppy-berries
Poppy-seeds
Poppy-grain
Stalk-of-the-Poppy

Reed-from-the-land-t'ahi-in-Asia
Female Reed

Saffron
Saffron-seeds
Blossom-of-the-Saffron

Seeds-from-the-Blossoms-of-the-Plants-of-the-Earth

Spring-plant

Sycamore-tree
Dough-of-the-Sycamore
Resin-of-the-Sycamore
Splinters-of-the-Sycamore
Milk-of-the-Sycamore
Milky-juice-of-the-Sycamore

Turpentine
Turpentine-nuts

Watermelon

Wheat
Grain-of-Wheat
Clean-Grain-of-Wheat
Green undried Wheat
Wheaten-flour

Willow-tree
Berry-of-the-Willow-tree
Splinters-of-the-Willow-tree

Wonderfruit
Seeds-of-the-Wonderfruit

Bread-of-the-Zizyphus-Lotus
Resin-of-the-Zizyphus-Lotus
Splinters-of-the-Zizyphus-Lotus
Wood-of-the-Zizyphus-Lotus

CHAPTER VII

ORGANIC REMEDIES

IF fancy played so large a part in the extraction of remedies from the plant and mineral world, it was in the domain of Organic therapeutics that were plumbed the depths of human credulity. Gods and Humans, Beasts, Birds, and Fishes, found their way into the pharmacopœia of Ancient Egypt. A poultice of Excrement-of-the-Gods is prescribed against tremors of the fingers. Human excrement mixed with Yeast-of-Sweet-Beer and Honey is recommended as a dressing for wounds. Male Semen is used as a flavouring agent in a mixture which relieves abdominal obstruction—by emesis, no doubt. Ass's Semen along with Rush-from-the-Green-Willow-tree, Fresh Bread, Herbs-of-the-Field, Figs, Grapes, and Wine cures the Great Debility, as also does another mixture composed of Excrement-of-the-adu-Bird and What-is-in-the-ut'ait-fruit, cooked in Olive Oil and Sweet Beer, and taken for four days. Man's Milk (reinforced it is true by Tortoise-shell, Granite, and Trash-from-the-Knife-Stone) cures the uases-abscess ; while as for the nesit-disease—

TO DRIVE OUT THE NESIT DISEASE

The-Two-Testicles-of-a-Black-Ass

Crush, rub in Wine, and let the Patient drink.

THE DISEASE DISAPPEARS AT ONCE.

But whether prescribed internally or externally many of the preparations confound all criticism. Imagine (if you can) a poultice consisting of the Zizyphus Lotus, Watermelon, Cat's dung, Sweet Beer, and Wine ; or a mixture of Rotten Flesh, Herbs-of-the-Field, and Garlic, cooked in Goose-oil and swallowed for four days against Debility ; or a Hair-restorer composed of Vulva, Phallus, and Black Lizard ; or a Hair-dye concocted of the Womb-of-a-Cat warmed in Oil with the Egg-of-the-gabgu-bird ; or another Hair-dye which combines a Tape-worm with the Hoof-of-an-Ass and the Vulva-of-a-Bitch ; or a mixture of Opium and Fly-dirt-which-is-on-the-Wall, to soothe a crying child ; or a Face-cream of Bullock's Bile and Ostrich Egg, beaten up with Fresh Milk ; or a diuretic of Water-from-the-Bird-Pond, Swill-of-Beer, and Fresh Milk ; or a purgative consisting of an Onion beaten up in Froth-of-Beer ; or a draught composed of the one-thirty-second part of the Tail-of-a-Mouse with Honey, one-third, for cooling the anus ; or another equally useful draught prepared by whipping up the Film-of-Dampness-which-is-found-on-the-Wood-of-Ships, in Froth-of-Beer, for Falling of the Womb ; or a mixture of Scrapings-of-a-Statue and Mint-of-the-Mountains, cooked in Oil and Wax, to be taken for four days to ' protect against everything.'

To compile an absolutely complete list of the

animal organic materia medica met with in the Papyrus would not be possible since (as with many of the plant and mineral substances) the identity of a considerable number of the animals mentioned is still beyond us. But even so the list of those animals whose identity is not in doubt, and who were called upon to sacrifice themselves in the cause of the Healing Art, is a formidable one as a glance at the following will show :

Lion
Hippopotamus
Crocodile
Ox
Cow
Calf
Mouse
Porcupine
Serpent
Tortoise
Lizard
Mole
Vulture
Bird-of-Passage
Swallow
Pigeon
Goose
Duck
Stag
Gazelle
Ram
Goat

Ass
Hog
Dog
Cat
Frog
Tadpole
Scorpion
Eel
Electric Eel
Crab
Swordfish
Ostrich
Locust
Tarantula
Beetle
Bat
Wasp
Fly
Tapeworm

As to the therapeutic substances which Ancient Egypt extracted from them, the list is, if anything, more startling still. They were forced to yield their

Hair
Feathers
Horns
Hoof
Hide
Eyes

Ears
Teeth
Brain
Blood
Bile
Bones
Marrow
Liver
Spleen
Guts
Uterus
Vulva
Phallus
Testicles
Semen
Fat
Tallow
Flesh
Shell
Wings
Excrement
Urine
Eggs
Milk
Toes
Tail

While both these lists are formidable ones it should be said that in many instances the physicians seem, all things considered, to have used a wise discretion in drawing upon them. Thus in the case of the Hog, although they used most of his body from his teeth to his testicles, they appear to have had the same contempt for his brain as is held nowadays, for nowhere is it prescribed. They also betrayed an acquaintance, amateurish perhaps, but still an acquaintance with psychology when they limited their Tortoise preparations to his brain, of which they knew so little, and his shell, of which they knew so much. The Porcupine was an animal which gave them another chance to display that uncanny sense of the fitness of things which we meet with here and there for they found use only for his quills, and then for the sole purpose of stimulating a bald scalp ; which, unless porcupines have changed unduly from that day, must have proved very stimulating indeed.

Amid such an assemblage it is gratifying to find the Ass, that never-failing friend of mankind throughout the ages, taking pride of place. For the relief of suffering humanity he sacrificed his blood, dung, ears, fat, head, hoof, jawbone, liver, milk, tallow, teeth, testicles, and semen. That equally faithful friend of man, the Cow, came a good second : she gave her bile, brain, blood, fat, flesh, horns, liver, milk, spleen, and tallow. And since it has already been noted that the gods contributed their excrement in the sacred cause, so it should also be noted that the humans contributed not only their excrement but their urine, their milk (both male and female !), and their semen (likewise both male and female !) in the same sacred cause.

Last, but not least, the Scribe himself. With

supreme audacity he imbued his own excrement and his urine, the very pen he wielded, the ink he used, and the papyrus he wrote upon, with Healing Magic, prescribing them as the spirit moved him against various infirmities and ills from threatened baldness to a distended bladder !

Chapter VIII

THE GODS AND THE HEALING ART

The gods of Egypt contribute to the compilation in a variety of ways. They are invoked collectively and individually to reinforce the curative effects of the remedies ; they are set down as the actual authors of some of the remedies ; and in one instance, as has been seen in a previous chapter, ' excrement of the gods ' is actually named as an ingredient of a compound designed to cure digital tremors.

It cannot be said that the Scribe is altogether flattering to the gods in his arrangement of the remedies attributed to them on Plate 46. The first of the remedies there quoted was, he informs us, compounded by the Great Ra himself who, it would appear, intended it as a sort of cure-all for all the ills of his own godly person. But it was a dismal failure as the entries that immediately follow show, for they are a series of remedies especially compounded by various lesser deities to cure the ills of this self-same Ra. Alas, their efforts were no more successful than those of Ra himself ; in fact all that they managed to achieve with *their* remedies was to give Ra a headache ! It now remained for a woman-doctor in the person of Isis to step into the breach and to set the August One on his feet again, not only curing him of his headache but relieving him as well of 'all sufferings and evils of any sort.'

ANOTHER REMEDY WHICH THE GODDESS ISIS PREPARED FOR THE GOD RA TO DRIVE OUT THE PAINS THAT ARE IN HIS HEAD :

Berry-of-the-Coriander	1
Berry-of-the-Poppy-plant	1
Wormwood	1
Berry-of-the-sames-plant	1
Berry-of-the-Juniper-plant	1
Honey	1

Make into one, mix with Honey, and smear therewith in order to make him well forthwith. When this remedy is used by him against all illnesses in the head and all sufferings and evils of any sort, he will instantly become well.

Among the lesser deities who prescribed for Ra was the goddess Tefnut, and to this female divinity must be accorded the honour of being the first woman-doctor to achieve the notice of history—even though her medical efforts only resulted in giving her divine patient a headache. But if a woman-doctor did give Ra a headache, we have seen that it was also a woman-doctor, Isis, who relieved him of that headache, thereby restoring the balance. Undoubtedly the success that attended the headache-cure compounded by Isis was due to the Opium it contained in the guise of Berry-of-the-Poppy-plant, and it may well be that it was her success with this drug that led that other woman-pioneer of medicine, Helen of Troy, in a later age to produce her nepenthe and to use it with the startling results that Homer records.

It is not to be wondered at then that the lengthy Invocation with which the Papyrus opens is addressed to Isis, and both here and elsewhere she is implored to impart healing powers to the remedies. Nowhere, it is well to point out, is the Magic Formula advocated as a cure *per se*, but it is an essential part of the treatment and without it the remedies might well be useless, and worse than useless. Together with the numerous Magic Formulæ scattered throughout the papyrus, the Invocation but serves to indicate the belief firmly held by the Ancient Egyptians that to effect the cure of disease it was first necessary to charm out of the body the evil spirit that had undoubtedly caused the mischief; then, by means of drugs, to repair the ravages he had caused during his temporary occupancy of the body. In the accompanying rendering of the opening Invocation the Rubrics of the Papyrus are represented by block letters, and it may be added the same applies wherever in this volume the actual text is quoted:

THE BEGINNING OF THE BOOK
ON THE PREPARATION OF MEDICINES
FOR ALL PARTS OF THE BODY OF A PERSON.

I came forth from Heliopolis with the priests of het-aat, the Lords of Defence, the Kings of Eternity and of Protection. I came forth from Sais with the

Maternal Goddesses who grant me protection. Words were given me by the Lord of the Universe wherewith to drive away the inflictions of all the gods, and deadly diseases of every sort.

SO MANY CHAPTERS ARE

on this my head, this my neck, these my arms, this my flesh, and these my limbs, to punish the scoffings of the High Ones who cause this disease to enter my flesh by working magic in these my limbs, so that as often as the disease penetrates into this my flesh, this my head, these my arms, into my body, and into these my limbs, Ra has compassion saying: I will protect him from his enemies. His leader, Hermes, it is who has given him the words, who provides the books, and who bestows upon the learned ones and on the physicians who follow him the glory of unravelling that which is obscure. Whom God loves, he quickens. I am one whom God loves, therefore he quickens me.

WORDS TO BE SPOKEN IN THE PREPARING OF MEDICINES FOR ALL PARTS OF THE BODY OF A PERSON WHO IS ILL.

As it is to be, a thousand times. This is the book for the healing of all diseases. May Isis heal me even as she healed Horus of all the pains which his brother Set had inflicted on him when he killed his brother Osiris! Oh Isis, thou great enchantress, heal me, deliver me from all evil, bad, typhonic things, from demoniacal and deadly diseases and pollutions of all sorts that rush upon me, as thou didst deliver and release thy son Horus! As I have penetrated into the Fire and have emerged from the Water, may I not fall into the snare of the day when I shall say: Little am I and piteous! Oh Ra, thou who hast spoken for thy body! Oh Osiris, thou who prayest for thy manifestation! It is Ra speaketh for his body; it is Osiris prayeth for his manifestation. Deliver me then from all possible evil, from bad, wicked, typhonic things, from demoniacal and deadly fevers of every sort.

SO MANY CHAPTERS THERE ARE TO SAY.

AS IT IS TO BE, A THOUSAND TIMES!

CHAPTER ON THE DRINKING OF MEDICINES.

Here follow the medicines. They come to drive away all sorts of things in this my heart, in these my limbs. The charms have great powers over the remedy. Once again. Do I not remember that Horus and Set were led to the great forecourt of Heliopolis to consult over the testicles of Set, and Horus became fresh as he was on earth? He does everything as he wills, as do those of the gods who are yonder. Words to be said when one drinks the medicines. As it is to be, a thousand times.

Chapter IX

DISEASES OF THE ALIMENTARY SYSTEM: CONSTIPATION, ETC.

A glance at the Papyrus Ebers dispels once for all any idea that Constipation is a scourge of the modern world brought about by modern conditions of living and eating. For page after page from the very beginning of the Papyrus the Scribe sets down purgative after purgative, all remedies designed to cure constipation or as he more crudely puts it 'to drive out the excrement in the body of a person.' Some of the preparations are to be drunk or eaten or chewed, some are to be made into pills and swallowed, others are to be formed into suppositories and inserted in the rectum. Castor Oil figures in not a few of them; unfortunately for the patients, in only one prescription is it the sole ingredient:

REMEDY TO CLEAR OUT THE BODY AND TO GET RID OF THE EXCREMENT IN THE BODY OF A PERSON

Berries-of-the-Castor-oil-tree	1

Chew and swallow down with Beer in order to clear out all that is in the body.

But they are not all as simple as that ; nor as effective, one may venture to add.

ANOTHER REMEDY FOR THE BODY

Leaves-of-the-Castor-oil-plant	$\frac{1}{4}$
Dates-of-the-Male-Palm	$\frac{5}{6}$
Cyperus-grass	$\frac{1}{16}$
Stalk-of-the-Poppy-plant	$\frac{1}{16}$
Coriander	$\frac{1}{16}$
Cold Beer	$\frac{1}{2}$

Keep moist, strain, and take for four days.

ANOTHER

Fresh Dates	I
Sea-salt	I
sebbet-juice	I

Mix in water, place in an earthenware receptacle, and put therein:

Crushed gengent-beans

Cook together, cover, and let the patient drink warm. Thereafter let him drink Sweet Beer.

REMEDY TO REGULATE EVACUATION

Honey	I
sasa-seeds	I
Wormwood	I
Elderberry	I
Berries-of-the-uan-tree	I
Kernel-of-the-ut'ait-fruit	I

Caraway	I
aaam-seeds	I
*X*am-seeds	I
Sea-salt	I

Form into a Suppository and put into the Rectum.

ANOTHER REMEDY TO DRIVE OUT THE DISEASED EXCREMENT IN THE BODY OF A PERSON

White-cake	I
Red tit-corn	I
Milk-of-a-Woman	

Mix into one and let the Person drink.

ANOTHER TO DRIVE OUT THE STERCORAL MASSES IN THE BODY

Figs	$\frac{1}{8}$
sebesten	$\frac{1}{8}$
Grapes	$\frac{1}{16}$
Caraway	$\frac{1}{64}$
Resin-of-Acanthus	$\frac{1}{32}$
Writing-fluid	$\frac{1}{64}$
Peppermint	$\frac{1}{32}$
gengent-beans	$\frac{1}{8}$
Sweet Beer	

Keep moist and take for four days.

Mass action may account for the efficacy of the foregoing remedies—if they were efficacious—but even this cannot be urged in favour of other of the remedies. Verdigris, even when ground up with Bread, made into three Pills, and swallowed down with Sweet Beer, does not sound very promising; neither does a mixture of Milk, Dough, and Honey, though it be taken for four days ; nor Elderberries and Honey cooked in Yeast-of-Beer-which-has-been-whipped-up ; nor a draught composed of Goose-grease and Lead-vitriol, flavoured though it be with Wine. And not even the emphasis of the Scribe convinces the impartial critic of the efficacy of another.

PREPARE THOU WELL THIS PURGATIVE.

HEREAFTER IT IS USED AGAINST THE CONSTIPATED BODY.

Herbs-of-the-Field	I
gengent-beans	I
aneb-plant	I
Bread-dough	I

Pound, make into one, make Four Cakes thereof, and let him eat.

Another remedy for Constipation which not only claims to act as a purgative but drives out all the diseases in the body, smacks more of a dawn-of-history cocktail than a purgative. It consists of Half-an-Onion mixed in Froth-of-Beer, and is further described as 'A DELIGHTFUL REMEDY AGAINST DEATH.' The remedy still persists in the shape of the 'life-saver' dispensed at the public bar, but the ingredients are no longer the same and its purgative action has long since disappeared.

The remedies for Constipation are appropriately followed by a succession of remedies 'to stop the diarrhœa.' As the following examples show their employment was purely empirical :

REMEDY TO STOP THE DIARRHŒA

Green Onions	$\frac{1}{8}$
Freshly-cooked-Gruel	$\frac{1}{8}$
Oil and Honey	$\frac{1}{4}$
Wax	$\frac{1}{16}$
Water	$\frac{1}{3}$ dena.

Cook and take for four days.

ANOTHER

Breadmeal	$\frac{1}{16}$
White-of-Egg	$\frac{1}{8}$
Onions	$\frac{1}{32}$
Water	$\frac{1}{3}$ dena.

Drink for four days.

ANOTHER

Breadmeal	$\frac{1}{16}$
Fresh Lead-earth	$\frac{1}{32}$
White-of-Egg	$\frac{1}{16}$
Water	$\frac{1}{3}$ dena.

Take for four days.

ANOTHER

Figs	$\frac{1}{8}$
Grapes	$\frac{1}{8}$

Bread-dough	$\frac{1}{32}$
pit-corn	$\frac{1}{32}$
Fresh Lead-earth	$\frac{1}{64}$
Onions	$\frac{1}{32}$
Elderberry	$\frac{1}{8}$

SING: O, HETU!
Again: O, HETU!

Which in the circumstances appears to be a very appropriate word to chant.

Chapter X

DISEASES OF THE ALIMENTARY SYSTEM: INDIGESTION, ETC.

Much as one may doubt the efficacy of the foregoing remedies in curing Constipation and in checking Diarrhœa, there can be no question as to one particular outcome of their employment, namely, Indigestion. Such a contingency, it is hardly necesssary to add, did not escape the Scribe and he offers a choice of twenty-one remedies for this condition. The chapter opens cautiously:

THE BEGINNING OF THE REMEDIES TO DRIVE AWAY INDIGESTION

Green Onions

Put in water in a new hunnu-glass and take for four days.

This for the Prohibitionists ; the Frothblowers were remembered in the next remedy.

ANOTHER

Onions

Cook in Sweet Beer and drink the third part thereof for four days.

If these failed it was, perhaps, due to their simplicity, a fault remedied in the following recipes.

ANOTHER

Take a Casserole, half-filled with Water, half with Onions. Let it stand for four days. See that it does not become dry. After it has stood moist, beat to a froth one-fourth of the third-part of the contents of this vessel, and let him who suffers from the vomiting drink it for four days so that he may become well immediately.

ANOTHER

Date-meal

Make into a dough in a hennu-vessel, put into two earthenware jugs, and set on the fire so that the dough cracks. When this has happened, put the pap in Fat and Olive Oil. To be eaten hot by the patient so that he may become well immediately.

Thereafter the Scribe panics. Having tried Onions and Dates separately he next prescribes them together, cooked in Milk. If this failed, as indeed it may have done, one could essay a sort of sundae prepared by crushing Wonderfruit in cooked Cow's Milk, and adding Cream to it. The dyspeptic with perverted cravings was not overlooked ; he was catered for with a sundae prepared by crushing Wild Lettuce in a sauce composed of Oil, Beer and Sour Milk, cooked together in a basin.

While much ink has been used up throughout the ages in setting down remedies upon remedies for Indigestion, it was only in Ancient Egypt that the ink-bottle itself was spilt into the remedy :

ANOTHER READY REMEDY TO DRIVE INDIGESTION OUT OF THE BODY

Figs	$\frac{1}{8}$
sebesten	$\frac{1}{8}$
Grapes	$\frac{1}{16}$
Caraway	$\frac{1}{64}$
Resin-of-Acanthus	$\frac{1}{32}$
Writing-fluid	$\frac{1}{64}$
Peppermint	$\frac{1}{32}$
gengent-beans	$\frac{1}{8}$
Sweet Beer	

Keep moist and take for four days.

Another remedy was probably intended for those victims of indigestion who complain of a stone-like feeling in the pit of the stomach :

ANOTHER

fut-ab-grain	I
meni-grain (an aromatic resin)	I
aam-plant	I

Crush into one. Take Seven Stones and make them hot in the fire. Take one of them and put therein the above-mentioned ingredients.

> Cover it up in a new vessel, bore a hole in its bottom (? lid), and thrust a calmus-reed through this hole. Put thy mouth to this reed that thou mayst inhale the steam therefrom. Likewise with the remaining six Stones. Afterwards eat something fatty, either Fat Meat or Oil.

But there is one remedy in particular that must be singled out for special mention:

ANOTHER REMEDY FOR INDIGESTION

> A Hog's Tooth
>
> Crush to powder, put inside four Sugar-cakes, and eat for four days.

A Hog's Tooth! What an inspiration! What an illustration of the habit of observation practised by these old-time medicos; for what is there on this earth that the tooth of a hog halts at on the score of indigestibility? Certainly this particular remedy is no longer in use among the best physicians, but it is still to the hog that the medical world looks to alleviate the pangs of Indigestion. All that *we* have done to improve on these pioneer organo-therapeutists is to powder his pancreas gland instead of his tooth, and to put it up in sugar-coated pills instead of the more clumsy sugar-cakes.

Sometimes the indigestion went further and resulted in inflammatory conditions of, and hardenings in, the abdomen. But whereas the former were treated by external remedies only, the latter were attacked both internally and externally. Some of the internal remedies were rather involved.

ANOTHER REMEDY FOR THE ABDOMEN

uah-grain	$\frac{1}{3}$
Grapes	$\frac{1}{3}$
Herbs-of-the-Field	$\frac{1}{4}$
Figs	a little
Sycamore-dough	
or Onions-from-the-Oasis.	

Crush and grind in Sweet Beer to which has been added the strength of the required herbs (also add Wheat and Barley Beer). Keep moist. Do not let it dry or a scum form thereover. Put thereto:

Honey	$\frac{1}{3}$
Goose-fat	$\frac{1}{3}$

Make into one and let the man or woman drink it.

But though involved, these mixtures were preferable to at least one external remedy:

ANOTHER TO DRIVE OUT THE HARDENING IN THE ABDOMEN

Bread-of-the-Zizyphus-Lotus	1
Cat's dung	1
Red-lead	1

Watermelon	I
Sweet Beer	I
Wine	I

Make into one and apply as a plaster.

A plaster that combines Cat's dung with Watermelon might be counted on to remove ' hardenings ' anywhere and in anybody.

The inflamed abdomen was not called upon to endure such indignities as these. The remedies were many, but two will suffice:

ANOTHER REMEDY TO DRIVE OUT INFLAMMATION IN THE ABDOMEN

A-piece-of-the-Stem-of-the-Flax-Plant	I
Fresh Milk	I

Apply to the abdomen of the Sick Person.

ANOTHER

Oil-from-the-Top-of-the-des-jar

Put on the Patient's abdomen.

None of the eight hundred remedies to be found in the Papyrus appear to have actually killed anyone of those whom they were intended to benefit. This is strange. But what is stranger still is that they did not prove fatal to every kind of parasite which lurked within the alimentary canal of the Ancient Egyptian. That they did not do so is clear from the remedies which are given to drive away these parasites, both

Roundworms and Tapeworms. The Roundworm was expelled by means of mixtures and draughts, two of the latter meriting commendation :

TO KILL THE ROUNDWORM

Bark-of-the-Pomegranate-root	1
Water	$\frac{1}{2}$

Keep moist, strain, and take for a day.

ANOTHER

Inner-of-the-Fruit-of-the-Caster-oil-tree	$\frac{1}{3}$
Yeast	$\frac{1}{3}$
Water	$\frac{1}{2}$

Keep moist, strain, and take for a day.

The Tapeworm proved more obstinate. Worm-cakes were recommended first. One cake was composed of Herbs-of-the-Field and Natron, baked into a cake with Cow's Bile. Another was compounded of Herbs-of-the-Field and Heart-of-the-mesa-Bird, along with Honey, Wine, and Sweet Beer. Or a draught could be used.

ANOTHER

Red-lead	1
gentet-plant, nes*x*i-corn, ta-bread	1
Petroleum	1
Sweet Beer	1

Stir, powder, strain, and take for one day.

And desperate cases could resort to a poultice:

TO DRIVE OUT THE DISEASES CAUSED BY THE TAPEWORM

Resin-of-Acanthus	I
Blossoms-of-the-Peppermint	I
Wild Lettuce	I
t'as-plant	I

Stir, mix into one, and apply as a poultice to the Body of the Man or Woman.

That some of the patients after a course of treatment on the lines indicated in the foregoing (and succeeding) pages should complain of anal discomfiture is not a thing for wonder. Consequently it occasions no surprise to find a large section devoted to relieving this *sequela*. As usual the thing was done thoroughly. Internal remedies were first prescribed:

REMEDY TO COOL THE ANUS

Onion-meal	$\frac{1}{32}$
Tail-of-a-Mouse	$\frac{1}{32}$
Honey	$\frac{1}{4}$
Water	$\frac{1}{3}$

Strain and take for four days.

A suppository was next recommended:

ANOTHER TO REDUCE THE SMARTING IN THE ANUS

Fat-of-the-Antilope	I
Caraway	I

Roll into a Pill and put in the Anus.

ANOTHER TO HEAL THE DISEASED ANUS

Cow-horn	1
Pieces-of-dried-Oil	1
Yeast-of-Wine	

Make a Peg (suppository) for the Man or Woman.

Next, bathing was advocated:

ANOTHER TO COOL AFTER THE OTHER MEDICINES

Ox-bile	$\frac{1}{3}$
Boiled Milk	$\frac{5}{6}$
Honey	$\frac{1}{3}$
Wonderfruit	$\frac{1}{2}$

Strain and pour on the anus for a day.

Finally if the anus refused to be cooled, and the smarting went a step further, a poultice was prescribed:

ANOTHER REMEDY AGAINST SORES IN THE ANUS

Egg-of-the-Goose	1
Guts-of-the-Goose	1

Clap on the anus.

Chapter XI

MINOR MEDICINE

Quite an appreciable amount of comfort may be derived from the fact that the Ancients of Egypt, wonderful as they were, yet groaned under the same petty annoyances that befall so many of us in this enlightened twentieth century, headaches, backaches, toe-aches, even corns, to mention a few. We find prescriptions for pains in the Head, the Bones, and the Trunk ; in the Backbone and the Joints ; in all the Limbs together and each of the Limbs separately ; in the Thigh, the Leg, even the Front-of-the-Shin, the Foot, and the Toes. But that is not all, for the Scribe, ever thorough, included a remedy for Corns, for Trembling-of-the-Fingers, for Tremors-of-all-the-Limbs, for a Squashed Leg, and for ' Tiredness in the Legs.' About the only ailment overlooked is ingrowing toe-nails ; but as it was in the pre-boot age (as we moderns know boots) perhaps they were not so much overlooked as unknown.

For the most part his Headache remedies are repulsive messes, their sole redeeming feature in our eyes being that they were not to be taken internally but rubbed in externally:

REMEDY TO DRIVE OUT THE PAIN IN THE HEAD

Inner-of-Onions	1
Fruit-of-the-am-tree	1
Natron	1
setseft-seeds	1
Bone-of-the-Sword-fish, cooked	1
Redfish, cooked	1
Skull-of-the-Crayfish, cooked	1
Honey	1
abra-ointment	1

Smear the Head therewith for four days.

For the stubborn headache there was a wide choice of other messy masses recommended for inunction. For instance, one could smear the aching head with an unguent composed of Hide-of-the-Hippopotamus and Poppy-seeds; or with another of Poppy-berries beaten up in Ass's Fat, to mention only two. Or there were various poultices and lotions. One consisted of Crocodile-earth beaten up with Egg-of-the-Ostrich; another of Mint-of-the-Mountains dissolved in Hippopotamus Oil along with Copper and Lead-vitriol; and still another of Ostrich Oil whipped up with Bile-of-the-Black-abdu-fish. But Aspirin has now displaced most, if not all, of these remedies in the public favour.

'For Pains in All the Limbs' the Scribe made a good start by instructing the Patient to mix up Castor Oil with Honey; but in the next few lines he spoilt everything by telling him to smear this all over the outside of his body instead of swallowing it and allowing it to do its work internally. Of course having got off the track at the start he found it impossible to right himself and accordingly went from bad to worse, his next effort being a poultice of Locusts which have been ground up in a mortar with Butter and Spices. For 'Pains in the Bones in Every Limb according to the Truth,' he recommended a poultice of Black Knife-stone with Fat, Honey, and Saltpetre as adjuvants. But according to the truth as we know it the use of Black Knife-stone, with or without Fat, Honey, and Saltpetre, in this connection is entirely fallacious, and not to be commended. The same can be said of the special poultice for the Thigh:

ANOTHER FOR THE THIGH

Bean-meal
Meal-of-the-pesen-bread
Sea-salt
Human Urine

Cook into one and apply as a Poultice.

And also for the Front-of-the-Shins, which was, however, let down more lightly:

REMEDY FOR THE FRONT OF THE SHINS

The Inner-of-the-Shadfish; what is found in its Head

Soak in Honey and apply as a Poultice.

IT WILL HEAL THE PATIENT FORTHWITH.

In the remedy for a Squashed Leg there are, some will see, the glimmerings of the first Bran Poultice:

ANOTHER FOR A SQUASHED LEG

Chopped-up Chaff soaked in Water

Lay thereon as a Poultice in order to heal him at once. It is also to be used for any Limb that thou wishest.

But diseased toes were a more formidable affair as the following shows:

TO HEAL THE DISEASED TOES

Fennel
Wax
Incense
Cyperus
Wormwood
Dried Myrrh
Poppy-plant
Poppy-grain
Elderberries
Berries-of-the-uan-tree
Resin-of-Acanthus
Dough-of-Acanthus
Resin-of-the-mafet-tree
Grain-of-Aloes
Fat-of-the-Cedar-tree
Fat-of-the-uan-tree
Fresh Olive Oil
Water-from-the-Rain-of-the-Heavens

Make into one and Poultice for four days.

It is rather late in the day, but no harm can be caused by proffering the suggestion that had the Diseased Toes been merely washed in Water-from-the-Rain-of-the-Heavens and then 'poulticed' with Fresh Olive Oil, the rest of the 'drugs' in this cumbersome remedy could have been discarded with advantage. However, Corns—as if to restore the balance—were dealt with simply. A poultice of various berries cooked in Cow-fat dispersed them.

The next two remedies are clearly directed against diseases of the nervous system, but since they deal with the effects of the disease on the limbs they are brought into this chapter:

TO DRIVE AWAY TREMBLINGS IN THE FINGERS

Incense
Caraway
Wax
Red-lead
Excrement-of-the-Gods
Honey
Figs
Fresh Lead-earth

Cook into one and apply as a Poultice.

TO DRIVE AWAY TREMBLINGS IN ALL THE LIMBS OF A PERSON

Fruit-of-the-Dompalm
Garlic
Honey

Copper
Verdigris

PUT A DOG'S HIDE ON HIM!
DO NOT PRESS THE HAND ON HIM!

Suppleness may also be dealt with here since it primarily affects the limbs. This attribute, if we take into consideration the remedies they were prepared to suffer to that end, must have been highly prized by the Ancients. The limbs could be made supple by smearing them with a liniment composed of Natron, Beans, Honey, Incense, and Sweet Myrrh, beaten up with Hippopotamus Oil, Crocodile Oil, Oil-of-the-Shadfish, Oil-of-the-adu-animal, and Oil-of-Two-Days. But the remedy *par excellence* for suppleness was Ass's dung. One simple remedy consisted of Ass's dung mixed with Honey and Sea-salt and smeared on the limbs. A more elaborate compound comprised Ass's dung, Honey, Figs, Date-juice, Sea-salt, Yeast-of-Wine, Bullock's Fat, Natron, Fresh tepu-grain, seneft-grain, and sesqa-grain; the whole being cooked and applied as a poultice.

'To make everything possible supple' they had a wide choice of salves. One salve consisted of Flesh-of-the-Shadfish and Honey beaten up in Yeast-of-Sweet-Beer. Another salve with surely more claim to colour than cure combined Writing-fluid, Vermilion, and Goat's Fat with Honey and several other ingredients, which were certainly only thrown in to make weight. In another salve Ass's dung reappears ; it is combined with Yeast-of-the-Opium-drink, Goat's Fat, Lettuce, Onions, Beans, and White Oil.

Sometimes it was a pathological cause such as 'Hardenings' which prevented the suppleness. In these cases the 'Hardenings' had first to be got rid of:

SALVE TO MAKE SUPPLE THE HARDENINGS

Hog's Fat
Oil-of-Worms
Oil-of-the-ab*x*ersu-animal
Mouse Oil
Cat's Oil

Gather into one and anoint therewith.

ANOTHER TO SOFTEN THE HARDENINGS

Fruit-of-the-Dompalm
Beans
Edelkraut
Fresh Milk
sebesten

CRUSH IT IN THE BIRD-OF-PASSAGE!
CRUSH IT IN ITS FEATHERS!

Apply as a Poultice.

Then once again, with that meticulous care which he displayed so often in his compilation, the Scribe rounds off the remedies with one by which the limbs 'could be protected against everything.' After mixing the Scrapings-from-a-Statue with Mint-of-the-Mountains and adding sasa-pieces, Oil, and Wax, one cooked the mixture, strained it (a not unnecessary precaution), and swallowed it for four days.

CHAPTER XII

MINOR SURGERY

SURGERY, judging by the Papyrus Ebers, was not a strong point with the Ancient Egyptians, and it is only when we wander through the domain of Major Surgery that we find the knife and the cautery advocated. Minor Surgery, what there is of it, is treated on ' bloodless ' lines.

A remedy ' to use against the Bite of a Crocodile ' is hardly the sort of entry which one would expect to see under the heading of Minor Surgery, but then times have changed. Three thousand years ago, we are forced to assume, bites from crocodiles were about as common as black eyes in these days; and to carry the simile still further, both were treated in the same way:

WHAT TO DO AGAINST THE BITE OF A CROCODILE

> If thou meetest a Crocodile's Bite, and thou findest his flesh equally fallen away on both sides, so thou coverest it with Raw Meat the first day.

A wound that merely demands a piece of raw meat to be clapped on it the first day could hardly be placed elsewhere than under Minor Surgery. Even a bite that one might suffer at the hands, or rather the teeth, of a lady or gentleman friend required more intensive treatment than that demanded by the bite of a crocodile:

REMEDY AGAINST THE BITE OR STING OF PEOPLE

Make thou for him a poultice of Raw Flesh on the first day. Afterwards treat him with Oil and Honey in order to do him good. Then put thou Oil in Wax in order to make him completely well at once.

Next, Burns. . . . Burns are troublesome lesions at the best of times and much needless suffering is saved if one can have at hand a quick and easy remedy to apply. The Ancients recognized this, although we might not be able to see any particular merit in the preparations they employed:

TO PREVENT BURN WOUNDS

A Frog

Warm in Oil and rub therewith.

ANOTHER

The Head-of-the-Electric-Eel

Warm in Oil and apply to the part of the body.

If one had more time there were other remedies that could be employed; for example, Elderberries and

Papyrus-plant mixed in Gum-water and applied thereto. Or, if one preferred a dry remedy:

ANOTHER

A-portion-of-Cake
Hair-of-a-Cat
Crush into one and apply thereto.

A more elaborate remedy, or series of remedies, is set forth for the use of those who wish to leave nothing to chance:

AGAINST BURNS: TO USE ON THE FIRST DAY

Black amat-juice
Put thereto.

ANOTHER ON THE FIRST DAY

Elderberries
uah-corn
Cat's dung
Mix into one in Cake-water and apply thereto.

TO USE ON THE SECOND DAY

Goat's dung
Burn, crush, rub in Yeast-that-is-fermenting, and put thereto.

TO USE ON THE THIRD DAY

Thorns-of-Acanthus, dried

Crush them in cooked durra-corn and Onions, put in Oil, and apply as a plaster.

TO USE ON THE FOURTH DAY

Wax

Roasted Cow's Fat

Palm-fibres

Make into one in uah-corn, and apply as a plaster.

TO USE ON THE FIFTH DAY

Onions

Red-lead

Fruit-of-the-am-tree

Crush, rub in Copper-splinters, make into one and apply as a plaster.

It is to their credit that these practitioners of a former day provided for emergencies, and in the unlikely event of a burn-wound going bad after the vigorous treatment set out above, a variety of formulæ existed. Thus, if the burn suppurated, a mixture of Elderberries, Papyrus-plant and Cat's dung, pounded in Cake-water, could be applied; or, if preferred, a mixture containing amongst other ingredients, Stone-from-the-Shore, Crocodile-incense, Fat-of-the-Egyptian-Goat, Onions, and Wax could be used. Or, again, Stone-from-the-Parting-of-the-Waters could be used instead of Stone-from-the-Shore in the last-mentioned prescription. If the burn still persisted in its downward course and began to 'turn white,' one is advised to use a remedy that, applied earlier in the day, one cannot help remarking, would have saved a deal of trouble; namely, a Linen-shirt steeped in Oil. Another simple remedy, although not so simple nor so effective as the foregoing must have proved, is, however, backed up by an unsolicited testimonial that is quite convincing in its brevity:

ANOTHER REMEDY TO DRIVE AWAY THE TURNING-WHITE OF A BURN

Durra-Bread-in-Oil-and-Salt

Mix into one and apply as a plaster in order that he may become well at once.

IT IS QUITE TRUE. I HAVE SEEN IT. IT HAS OFTEN HAPPENED TO ME.

But, as every medical man knows, Burns can be stubborn affairs. Hence it is not surprising that in spite of the above unsolicited testimonial the Ancients found some burns beyond the ingenuity of mortal man, and were forced to invoke the aid of the gods to reinforce the therapeutic effect of the remedies:

INCANTATION FOR A BURN

'O son, Horus! There is Fire in the Land! Water is not there and thou art not there! Bring Water over the River-bank to quench the Fire.'

To be spoken over Milk-of-a-Woman-who-has-Borne-a-Son.

ANOTHER INCANTATION FOR A BURN

'O thou son of god, Horus! There is Fire in the Land! Though there be water there or not now, the Water is in thy Mouth, the Nile is at thy Feet when thou comest to quench the Fire.'

To be spoken over Milk-of-a-Woman-who-has-Borne-a-Son.

Cake

Ram's Hair

Apply to the Burn.

The victim of a Burn had little to thank the Healing Profession for, it will be admitted; but the person unfortunate enough to contract an open wound had still less. One remedy directs that Cow's Fat or Cow's Flesh be placed on the wound in order to ripen (i.e., decompose) it; after which it is treated with a variety of Fats, Oil, and Fruits, and finally with a plaster of Powder-of-Fresh-Ivory mixed in Honey. But worse was to follow:

ANOTHER REMEDY TO DRESS A WOUND

Human excrement

Crush in Yeast-of-Sweet-Beer, sefet-oil, and Honey, and apply as a Poultice.

If there be any who still complain of the slowness of medical progress, let him be thankful that in the extraction of splinters, to mention another department, we have advanced since the days of Tut-Ankh-Amen. It does not seem much to boast of, and yet. . . .

WHAT TO DO TO DRAW OUT SPLINTERS IN THE FLESH

The per-baibait-bird-with-Honey

Apply thereto.

ANOTHER

Worms' blood, cook and crush in Oil;
Mole, kill, cook, and drain in Oil;
Ass's dung, mix in Fresh Milk

Apply to the opening.

ANOTHER

Male-and-Female-Semen

Apply thereto.

ANOTHER

Skull-of-the-Shadfish, cooked in Oil

Apply to the point of the splinter. Thereby it comes out.

ANOTHER

Incense
Dough
Sea-salt
Wasp's dung
Fat

Red-lead
Wax

Apply thereto. It draws the matter thereout.

It is unfortunate that the Scribe did not think it worth while to describe the 'uases' abscess so that we might make an effort to identify it. That it was a stubborn eruption, the remedies show. One that cures the abscess by 'making the blood fall' is composed of Man's Milk, Granite, Tortoise-shell, and Trash-from-the-Knifestone. Just as picturesque, and assuredly as useless, is the second remedy:

ANOTHER REMEDY AGAINST THE UASES ABSCESS

Blood-of-a-Dove
Blood-of-a-Goose
Blood-of-a-Swallow
Blood-of-a-Vulture

Anoint therewith.

'Stinking ulcers'—their number must have been legion—were dealt with at length, but why the tag of advice was attached only to the following remedy is somewhat puzzling. It could with advantage have been appended to many others in the Papyrus:

ANOTHER REMEDY TO DRIVE OUT A STINKING ULCER IN THE BODY OF A MAN OR WOMAN

Egg-of-an-Ostrich
Tortoise-shell

Thorns-of-the-am-tree

Warm and anoint therewith.

BUT DON'T GET TIRED DOING IT!

To dry a wound it was plastered with Incense, Onions, and Cow Fat; or if the only animal available was a goat, then some Goat's Fat was beaten up with Onions and Wax and used as a poultice. For those who had any objection to Cows or Goats there remained the Hippopotamus and the Wasp, not to mention the Hog:

ANOTHER TO HEAL

Refuse-of-durra

Mix in Fat-of-the-Hippopotamus, or of the Hog, and apply as a poultice.

ANOTHER

Dough
Incense
Tooth-grain
Wasp's dung
Red-lead
Salt-from-the-North
Wax

Crush and put thereon.

Wheals, the result of blows, are curtly dismissed with a draught, a poultice, and a salve. Slaves were lucky to get that much consideration:

REMEDY TO DRIVE AWAY THE WHEALS FROM BLOWS

Honey
Cow's Brain
Mason's Clay
Linseed-water
Date-juice

Cook, and apply as a plaster.

ANOTHER

Dust-of-Alabaster
Dust-of-a-Statue
Granite
Fresh Milk

Anoint therewith.

ANOTHER

A portion-of-hemit, dried

Crush, powder, and put in a Sugar-cake. One-part thereof soaked in Honey to be eaten by the person.

Skin-grafting, it may be shortly said, formed no part of the accomplishments of the medical practitioner in Ancient Egypt. Nevertheless he did his best to stimulate granulation:

TO MAKE THE FLESH GROW

Collyrium
Cow-fat

Chips-of-Verdigris
Honey
Crush, and apply as poultice.

Curiously enough this remedy appeared to have succeeded at times; in fact to have over-succeeded on occasions, for it is followed by another remedy to check excessive granulation. Since this, however, was composed of an unguent concocted of Ostrich-egg ground down with Tortoise-shell and Thorns-of-the-am-tree, its efficacy may be seriously doubted.

Chapter XIII

THE URINARY SYSTEM

The Urinary System received nothing like the detailed attention paid to the Alimentary System. But it made up for that in variety. Urinary troubles in the adult were corrected in three ways: a rectal injection of Olive Oil, Honey, Sweet Beer, Sea-salt, and Seeds-of-the-Wonderfruit was one way. Anointing the Phallus was another:

TO REGULATE THE URINE

*X*et-plant

Mix in Fresh Milk and apply to the Phallus.

ANOTHER

Crocus-from-the-South	1
Beans, roasted	1

Put in Oil and anoint the Phallus therewith.

ANOTHER

Wood-of-the-Zizyphus-Lotus

Mix in Yeast-of-the-mesta-drink, and anoint the Phallus therewith.

A third method was by means of mixtures:

REMEDY TO REGULATE THE URINE

A-measuring-glass-filled-with-Water-from-the-Bird-pond	1
Elderberry	1
Fibres-of-the-asit-plant	1
Fresh Milk	1
Beer-Swill	1
Flowers-of-the-Cucumber	1
Green Dates	1

Make into one, strain, and take for four days.

The less said about the remedies for the treatment of Polyuria and frequency of Micturition the better. But it is to the credit of Egypt's surgeons that they did not practise urethral dilatation in cases of stricture. Instead, the obstruction was treated on medical lines.

REMEDY TO FORCE OUT THE URINE

Crocus-from-the-Hills	$\frac{1}{4}$
Crocus-from-the-Delta	$\frac{1}{8}$
abu-plant-from-Upper-Egypt	$\frac{1}{16}$
abu-plant-from-Lower-Egypt	$\frac{1}{16}$
Berry-of-the-uan-tree	$\frac{1}{16}$
Fresh Gruel	$\frac{1}{8}$
Linseed	$\frac{1}{16}$
uam-seeds	$\frac{1}{16}$

duat-plant	$\frac{1}{16}$
Water	$\frac{1}{16}$

Keep moist, strain, and take for four days.

Urinary ailments in children were specially prescribed for. To regulate Micturition in a child a Blossom-plucked-from-the-nebat-plant was put in Sweet Beer. If a girl, she had to drink the mixture out of a cool flask. If a boy, he had to drink it out of a hennu-vessel. A quaint remedy relieved retention in a child:

REMEDY FOR A CHILD FOR CLEARING OUT THE ACCUMULATION OF URINE IN HIS BODY

An-old-Book-cooked-in-Oil

Smear on his Body.

An old Book means, of course, a discarded papyrus and in this case the virtue of the papyrus would be enhanced by the writing-fluid, both of which 'drugs'—paper and ink—are as much a part of the pharmacopœa of the day as Red-lead or Honey, or a host of others, and are frequently prescribed for many ailments.

Another remedy proposed for a child who is having trouble with his urine must be noticed here. *X*ent-grains are made into a pill, which is given to the child in his food if he is old enough to manage it. But, if it is a suckling that is to be treated, the wet-nurse is directed to warm it in her mouth first, and then to spit it into the mouth of the babe for four days. This interpretation of the passage, however, is open to question and is opposed by several writers who have quoted the prescription in their works. Their contention is that the Scribe intended the mother to swallow the Pill, the child receiving the benefit of it in the maternal milk.

Chapter XIV

DISEASES OF WOMEN

The women's section covers some four or five pages of the Papyrus and includes remedies for errors of menstruation and lactation, diseases of the breasts and genitalia, aids to abortion and parturition, and various valuable hints to nursing mothers. Two of these hints enable them to distinguish the quality of their milk: thus, if the milk be good, it smells like the pollen of uah-grain; if, on the other hand, the milk be bad, it smells like the entrails of the mehit-fish. Other hints enable them to prognosticate the fate of the new-born child:

PROGNOSIS FOR A CHILD ON THE DAY IT IS BORN

If it cries ni, it will live.
If it cries ba, it will die.

ANOTHER

If it lets a loud lamentation be heard, it will die.
If it looks down its face it will thereupon die.

To regulate menstruation the patient was douched with a mixture of Garlic and Wine. If this failed, a douche composed of Fennel, Wonderfruit, Honey and

Sweet Beer was substituted and persisted in for four days. To protect a virgin from Leucorrhœa it was necessary to anoint her breast, body, and all the limbs with a lotion prepared by crushing the dried liver of a Swallow in Sour Milk.

To produce Milk in the breast of a woman about to suckle a child, Bones-of-the-Swordfish were warmed in Oil and her backbone smeared therewith. The same result could be brought about by mixing Fragrant Bread (which had been made from Soured Durra) with the Poppy-plant, and making her eat it while she sat cross-legged.

To bring about abortion, only one remedy is given: Dates, Onions, and the Fruit-of-the-Acanthus, were crushed in a vessel with Honey, sprinkled on a cloth, and applied to the Vulva. It ensured abortion either in the first, second or third period. To hurry on labour, however, there was no lack of remedies:

REMEDY TO CAUSE A WOMAN TO BE DELIVERED

Peppermint

Let the woman apply it to her bare posterior.

ANOTHER TO CAUSE ALL AND EVERYTHING THAT IS IN THE BODY OF A WOMAN TO FALL

Pot-of-a-new-hennu-vessel

Crush in Warm Oil and pour on her genitals.

ANOTHER TO LOOSEN A CHILD IN THE BODY OF A WOMAN

Sea-salt

Clean Grain-of-Wheat
Female Reed

Plaster the abdomen therewith.

ANOTHER

Fresh Salt
Honey

Strain and take for one day.

ANOTHER

Fennel
Incense
Garlic
sert-juice
Fresh Salt
Wasp's dung

Make into a ball and put in the Vagina.

ANOTHER

Tail-of-a-Tortoise
Shell-of-a-Beetle
sefet-oil
sert-juice
Oil

Crush into one and poultice therewith.

To remedy a diseased Breast one could plaster it for four days with a compound of Calamine, Cow's Brain, and Wasp's dung ; or one could invoke the goddess Isis by means of a magic formula:

MAGIC FORMULA FOR THE BREAST

The Breast is the same diseased Breast of Isis who in the city of *X*ebt bore the gods Su and Tefnut!

She has prepared for it this Magic Formula to be said over aat-plant, Health-corn, over the Fruitful-Part-of-Reeds, over the Hair-of-the-abt-plant, which we bring here to drive out all kinds of Deadly Diseases, as many as there are, cleansing by a discharge in the Left Side.

Prepare it against all kinds of Deadly Diseases. Neither express, nor rub, nor bleed. Prevent the dryness of the Eyes which ensues.

SPEAK OVER AAT-PLANT, OVER HEALTH-GRAINS, OVER THE-FRUITFUL-PART-OF-REEDS, OVER HAIR-OF-THE-HEAD-OF-THE-ABT-PLANT.

LET IT POUR OUT ON THE LEFT SIDE.

MAKE SEVEN PORTIONS AND GIVE THEM.

The Vulva could be protected against the entry of disease by injecting a douche in which Garlic and Horn-of-a-Cow figure as ingredients. Should this prophylactic fail and inflammation ensue, the douche was changed to one of Bile-of-the-Cow, Cassia, and Oil. If the disease progressed and corrosion occurred, the Cow was discarded for the Hog, and a douche of Fresh Dates and Hog's Bile administered. If, in spite of these vigorous measures, pustules appear in the vagina, recourse is now had, as so often before, to the Ass, and the douche is composed of Fresh Dates and Ass's Milk.

To correct the displaced uterus, the remedies recommended were almost as ingenious as they were useless:

REMEDY TO ALLOW THE WOMB OF A WOMAN TO SLIP INTO ITS PLACE

The-Film-of-Dampness-which-is-found-on-the-Wood-of-Ships (mould)

Rub in Yeast-of-Fermented-Beer and let her drink it.

ANOTHER

Put an Ibis-of-Wax on the coals and allow the fumes thereof to penetrate into her sex-organs.

ANOTHER

Dried Human excrement

Put in Incense; the woman bends herself over the same and lets the fumes thereof penetrate into her sex-organs.

ANOTHER

Oil-of-the-Earth (? Petroleum) with peddu (manure)

Keep in Honey and rub the body of a woman therewith.

ANOTHER

Dried Excrement
Froth-of-Beer

Rub the finger of the woman therewith and put it to all her limbs against her sufferings. (Joachim suggests that she was to smear the prolapsed uterus.)

With one more extract from the women's section we may pass on:

When thou examinest a woman who has lived many years without her Menstruation having appeared; she vomits something like foam and her body is as though a fire were under it, but she recovers after the vomiting; then say thou to her: This is a rising of Blood to the Womb. So soon as she has spoken the Magic Formula, and has had coitus, make thou for her:

Berry-of-the-uan-tree	$\frac{1}{32}$
Caraway	$\frac{1}{64}$
Incense	$\frac{1}{64}$
uah-grain	$\frac{1}{16}$

Put Cow's Milk to the Fire with Thigh-tallow. Add Milk thereto and let her take for four days.

Chapter XV

DISEASES OF THE SKIN

'Skins,' we gather from the remedies prescribed, were placed in three categories : irritative, exfoliative, and ulcerative. For the common Itch a mixture composed of Onion, crushed in Honey and taken in Beer, was prescribed. If the Itch was confined to the Neck, a Chopped-up Bat applied to it as a poultice healed it 'at once.' For the Thigh :

REMEDY FOR THE THIGH

Onions
Dried Beans
Red Natron
Sea-salt
Sour Milk

Make into a poultice.

It heals at once.

If the itching spread to all the limbs and became generalized, various remedies were available. Among them a Poultice of Corn, Natron, Clay-from-the-Gate, Onions, Incense, and Refuse-of-Dates. This was calculated to soothe it, but there was also a certain-sure remedy for it:

ANOTHER TO ALLAY ITCHING

Cyperus-from-the-Meadow
Onion-meal
Incense
Wild Date-juice

Make into one and apply to the scurvy place.

LOOK TO IT BECAUSE THIS IS THE TRUE REMEDY.
IT WAS FOUND AMONG THE PROVEN REMEDIES IN THE TEMPLE OF THE GOD, OSIRIS.
IT IS A REMEDY WHICH DRIVES AWAY THE SCURF IN EVERY LIMB OF A PERSON.
YES, IT HEALS AT ONCE.
YOU SEE.

If the itching were accompanied by ' blood corrosion ' the trouble became involved, and mild or simple remedies were out of the question. A concoction of Elderberries, Linseed, Wormwood, Natron, and various native plants, rubbed in Semen-of-a-Man, Yeast-of-Wine, and Juice-of-the-Wild-Date, was warmed and applied as a poultice. In the event of this and similar remedies not bringing relief, rectal injections were employed. One such enema consisted of Fresh Milk and Sea-salt ; another of Fresh Milk, Sea-salt, and Incense ; another of Urine, Onions, and Oil ; and still another of Honey, Fresh Milk, Olive Oil, Copper-rust, and Collyrium. This line of treatment is that known as counter-irritation and persists to this day, though not in this form, nor with these (nor similar) remedies, nor indeed for this particular disease.

For common scurf the ketket-plant and the Berry-of-the-uan-tree were ground into one with the Milk-of-a-Woman, strained, and drunk for four days. A simpler but hardly less pleasant remedy comprised equal parts of Sea-salt and Beer, which likewise had to be taken for four days. If the scurf was complicated by ' Hardenings in all the Limbs of a Person,' heroic measures in the shape of a poultice composed of Pieces-of-excrement, Cat's dung, Dog's dung, and Berries-of-the-*X*et-plant were taken. ' IT DRIVES OUT ALL THE SCURF,' the Scribe added reassuringly. One devoutly hopes so.

Further heroic measures were employed, or recommended, when ' Scabs in every Limb ' appeared. First an endeavour was made to coax them away with a poultice of Clay-from-the-Wall, Wheaten Flour, and Fat-of-the-deher-animal, strained into Yeast-of-Sweet-Beer. If they resisted this, another poultice was at hand: Cyperus-from-the-Marshes, Cyperus-from-the-Fields, Cyperus-knots, and Red Corn, were crushed in Fresh Oil, Goose-oil, and Semen. But even this failed on occasion, for other remedies followed:

ANOTHER

huru-grain in Men's Milk.

Put on the Ulcer until it falls off.

ANOTHER

Ass's Milk
am of dough

Put on the Ulcer until it falls off.

ANOTHER

Wasp's dung in Milk-of-the-Sycamore.

Put on the Ulcer until it falls off.

Only half of the good work was accomplished however when the scabs had fallen off, for the lesions were now assailed with any of the following :

AFTER IT HAS FALLEN OFF PUT THEREON

Scribe's excrement.

Mix it thoroughly in Fresh Milk and apply as a Poultice.

ANOTHER

Tops-of-the-Cedar-tree.

Mix with Milk-of-a-Woman-who-has-borne-a-Son, and apply as a Poultice.

ANOTHER

Wasp's dung
Fresh Milk

Put thereon.

ANOTHER

A piece of Lead
Cat's dung
Dog's dung

Apply as a Poultice.

ANOTHER

A Hog's Tooth
Cat's dung
Dog's dung
aau-of-samu-oil
Berries-of-the-*x*et-plant

Pound and apply as a Poultice.

'To drive out a Stinking Ulcer either in a Man or Woman' one rubbed the body with a ball made of Powdered Onions. A Paste was also provided:

ANOTHER

Ostrich Egg
Tortoise-shell
Thorns-of-the-am-tree

Warm and anoint therewith.

BUT DON'T GET TIRED DOING IT.

If one did 'get tired doing it' there was still another remedy. This was of the cure-all kind:

REMEDY TO FREE THE FLESH FROM DISEASE

Ass's Milk
Resin-of-Acanthus
Indigo
duat-plant
Turpentine-nuts
Honey

Cook, strain, and take for four days.

To drive away leprous spots on the skin, one cooked some Onions in a mixture of Sea-salt and Urine and applied it to the spots. Herpes on the face was treated by a frequent dressing of the Inner-part-of-the-Castor-Oil-tree and Red-lead, the rouge effect of the latter probably accounting for its inclusion. But Eczema-of-the-Head was not to be dismissed so lightly. In fact it was particularly troublesome. On the first day the head was painted with a ' lotion ' of durra-meal and Fruit-of-the-Dompalm, warmed in Soft Fat, and was then bound up. On the second day the head was anointed with Fish-oil. On the third day with Hippopotamus Oil. On the fourth day with abra-oil. After this course of intensive treatment the offending head, if the Eczema still persisted, was smeared daily with Bread-meal and dressed with ' Rotted Cereals.'

Chapter XVI

DISEASES OF THE EYES

Nine pages of the original papyrus are devoted to eye-conditions, a fact which need occasion no surprise to anyone acquainted with that country even after the thousands of years that separate us from that far-distant period. In a separate volume published in 1889 Ebers gave a detailed translation of this interesting chapter, differentiating the following conditions:

Blepharitis
Blindness
Carcinoma
Cataract
Chalazion
Chemosis
Ectropion
Entropion
Granulation
Hæmorrhage
Hydrophthalmus
Inflammation
Iritis
Leucoma
Ophthalmoplegia

Pinguecula
Pterygium
Staphyloma
Trichiasis

To improve the sight a 'lotion' prepared by warming Chips-of-a-new-hennu-pot in Fresh Milk was recommended. Another lotion could be prepared by combining Cream with the Milk-of-a-Woman-who-has-borne-a-Son. Apply to the eyes frequently, is added. A number of salves are also given in each of which Collyrium figures. Thus in one the Collyrium is simply combined with Honey; in another with Honey and Sap-from-Fresh-Onions; in another with the Marrow-of-an-Ox; in another with Goose-grease and Water; in another with Incense and Real Lapis lazuli; in another with Antimony, Copper-vitriol, Writing-fluid, and Onions; and in still another with Writing-fluid, Myrrh, Opal-resin, Arabian-wood-powder, and Saltpetre-from-Upper-Egypt.

For Bleary Eyes one beat up Myrrh, Onions, Verdigris, and Cyperus-from-the-North, with Antilope-dung, Clear Oil, and Entrails-of-the-qadit-animal. This could be painted on with a Vulture's feather. Fortunately for Bleary-eyed panel patients of that day, and for those whose means did not run to Antilopes and Vultures (not to mention qadit-animals) the homely Ass—as so often before—stepped into the breach and offered himself, or rather part of himself, for their benefit:

ANOTHER REMEDY

> Ass's Tooth
>
> Mix in Water and apply around the Patient's eyes so that he recovers quickly.

The remedy does not sound very convincing but it has the merit of being clean and as such is infinitely to be preferred to the 'remedy' employed by a recent patient of the writer who for the three weeks preceding had been vigorously (and to his surprise unavailingly) bathing his bleary eyes, night and morning, with his own urine!

A simple poultice of Incense and Crocus, equal parts, often sufficed to clear up Bloodshot Eyes. If it did not a more complicated poultice composed of Onions, Verdigris, Collyrium, and Arabian-wood powder, crushed 'to a powder' with Ink and Water was recommended. Then there was another:

ANOTHER TO DRIVE OUT BLOOD IN THE EYES

> Two Clay vessels: in one put powdered Fruit-of-the-Dompalm and Milk-of-a-Woman-who-has-borne-a-Son. In the other Cow's Milk. Keep moist. In the morning bathe both eyes from the Fruit-of-the-Dompalm. Next wash the Eyes with the Cow's Milk four times for six days.

Xanthelasma seemingly proved a troublesome condition, for after laying down various remedies the

Scribe thought it advisable to impart some ginger into the treatment:

ANOTHER TO DRIVE OUT FAT-IN-THE-EYES

Red-lead	I
Goose-grease	I

Smear the eyes therewith.

SEE TO IT!

Another remedy approximated more to the modern treatment of the disease:

ANOTHER TO DRIVE OUT FAT-IN-THE-EYES

Knife-stone

Mix in Fresh Milk and apply thereto very often.

To-day it is the Knife instead of a Knife-stone that we apply to the eye, while the patient is instructed to drink the Fresh Milk.

'To him whose two eyes suffer from a flow of matter' a poultice of Clay-from-a-Statue, Leaves-of-the-Castor-oil-tree, and Honey, is advised. To restore the lustre of the eyes one could apply a poultice of Onions, Resin, and Verdigris, crushed in the Milk-of-a-Woman-who-has-borne-a-Son. If a film covered the eyes the remedies were many, but two will suffice:

TO DISPEL THE FILM IN THE EYES ON THE FIRST DAY

Water-from-the-Bird-pond	I

Whether this was drunk or merely applied to the eyes does not appear; but fortunately in the next remedy there was no room for doubt:

ANOTHER REMEDY FOR THE FILMING-OVER WHICH RISES IN THE EYE

Dried-excrement-from-the-Body-of-a-Child	1
Honey	1

Put in Fresh Milk and then apply to the Eyes.

Leucoma was a complaint that set these far-off Oculists on their mettle. They tried to coax it away with a lotion of Cream and Milk, or another of Collyrium, Ink, and Water. These failing they ground some Ebonywood and Collyrium to powder and applied it. Next they dressed the eyes with a poultice of Powdered Granite. Then getting desperate they tried a 'paste' made from Collyrium and the Bile-of-the-abdu-fish. Finally they resorted to Magic, plus the Brain-of-a-Tortoise mixed with Honey:

ANOTHER TO DRIVE OUT THE WHITE GROWTH IN THE EYES

There is a Shouting in the Southern Sky in the Darkness.
There is an Uproar in the Northern Sky.
The Hall of Pillars falls into the Waters.
The Ship-folk of the Sun-god beat their oars so that the heads at his side fall into the water.
Who leads hither what he finds?

I lead forth what I find.
I lead forth your heads.
I lift up your necks.
I fasten what has been cut from you in its place.
I lead you forth to drive away the God of Fevers and all possible Deadly Arts.

So MANY THERE ARE.

A formula to repeat over the Brain-of-a-Tortoise that is mixed in Honey, and then laid on the Eyes.

Cataract was another condition which had the Ancients at their wits' end. Goose-grease and Honey was tried as a poultice; Isinglass and Verdigris; Lapis lazuli, Milk, Incense, and Crocodile-earth. But how intractable this disease must have proved itself is revealed in the call made to the gods to reinforce the remedy:

ANOTHER TO DRIVE OUT CATARACT IN THE EYES

Come, Verdigris!
Come, Verdigris!
Come, Thou Fresh One!
Come, Efflux from the Eye of the god Horus!
It comes, That which issues forth from the Eye of Tum!
Come, Juice that gushes from Osiris!
He comes to him, he drives away from him Water,

Matter, Blood, Inflammation of the Eyes,
Mattery-discharge, Blindness, Dripping Eyes.

This the God of Fever works all Deadly Arts, the uxedu of every kind, and all things evil of these eyes.

So many there are of them.

Words to be spoken over Verdigris mixed with Beetle-wax.

Add Cyperus thereto and carefully apply to the Eye.

Another growth in the eye, Pterygium, was not looked on kindly, judging by the remedies which these people appeared ready to submit to. Certainly the Scribe leads off with an inoffensive poultice of Honey-comb, following it with another of Beetle-wax, but these must have proved useless for he soon passes on to more complicated and stronger remedies. Excrement-of-the-henut-bird, is recommended, mixed up with Sea-salt and Incense; then descending from the clouds he sets down another composed of Lizard's dung, Collyrium, Soda-from-Upper-Egypt, and Honey. Another poultice is composed of Black Knife-stone and Crocodile-earth, mixed up with Honey and flavoured with Incense. He made an attempt at a golden-eye ointment, too, when he crushed some Collyrium in the Egg-of-a-Vulture; but what the colour of the following turned out to be only a brave man would say:

ANOTHER TO DRIVE OUT PTERYGIUM

Red-lead	1
Powdered-wood-from-Arabia	1
Iron-from-Apollonopolis-parva	1
Calamine	1
Egg-of-an-Ostrich	1
Saltpetre-from-Upper-Egypt	1
Sulphur	1
Honey	1

Make into one and apply to the Eyes.

Eyes which suffered from a 'flow of matter' were dismissed with a mere couple of remedies. Clay-from-a-Statue was ground up in Honey along with some Leaves-from-the-Castor-Oil-tree, and applied to the eyes. The second remedy was not so easily put up. Some Real Collyrium was soaked in Water for four days; then for another four days it was soaked in Goose-grease. It was now washed in the Milk-of-a-Woman-who-had-borne-a-Son, and allowed to dry for nine days. Thereafter it was crushed with some Myrrh, made up into a ball, and rubbed on the eye.

The victims of ingrowing eyelashes must have been a veritable godsend to the rising ophthalmologist in Ancient Egypt. At the same time they must have proved a very severe drain on the live-stock of the country, as may be seen from a perusal of some of the remedies prescribed for that irritating affliction:

TO DRIVE OUT TRICHIASIS

Myrrh	1
Lizard's Blood	1
Bat's Blood	1

Tear out the Hairs and put thereon in order to make him well.

TO PREVENT THE HAIR GROWING INTO THE EYE AFTER IT HAS BEEN PULLED OUT

Incense-ground-in-Lizard's-dung	1
Cow's Blood	1
Ass's Blood	1
Pig's Blood	1
Dog's Blood	1
Stag's Blood	1
Collyrium	1
Incense	1

Crush, rub into one in the different kinds of Blood, and place on the part whence the Hair has been pulled out so that it may not grow again.

ANOTHER

Bat's Blood	1
Rim-of-a-new-hennu-vessel	1
Honey	1

Powder and place where the Hair has been pulled out.

ANOTHER

Fat-of-an-Ox	1
Olive Oil	1
Entrails-of-Moles	1

Crush into one, put on the fire, and put in the place of the Hair.

ANOTHER

Brain-of-the-uuat-bird	1

Smear a Vine-leaf therewith and put in the place whence the Hair has been pulled out.

ANOTHER

Wasp's dung	1
Red-lead	1
Urine	1

Mix and put in the places where the Hair has been pulled out.

Still another eye-condition which set these Ancients thinking was Blindness. Only three remedies were given for this calamity. The first, a 'lotion' made by crushing Dried Myrrh in Sour Milk, we may be sure accomplished nothing. The second, however, a poultice of Powdered Onions, most assuredly made the blind man see stars. The third remedy spared the patient somewhat, the disease being attacked through that less-sensitive organ, the ear:

ANOTHER AGAINST BLINDNESS

The Two Eyes of a Pig; remove the water therefrom
True Collyrium
Red-lead
Wild Honey

Crush, powder, make into one, and inject into the Ear of the Patient. Thereby he will at once recover. When thou hast seen properly to this mixing, repeat this Magic Formula:

I HAVE BROUGHT THIS THING AND PUT IT IN ITS PLACE. THE CROCODILE IS WEAK AND POWERLESS.
(Twice).

'For the Drawing-together of the Pupil of the Eye,' whatever that may mean, one bathed the eye frequently with a lotion made by crushing Shavings-from-Ebony-Wood with Soda-from-Upper-Egypt in Water. For a swelling in the Nose caused by inflammation of the tear-sac a salve composed of Collyrium, Dried Myrrh, Arabian-wood powder, and Honey, was rubbed in for four days. 'MARK THIS WELL (the Scribe adds), FOR IT IS THE RIGHT THING TO DO.' Another eye-salve is prescribed for 'Driving out Tumours in-the-Head,' while the Scribe also finds room to quote two salves for general use: one 'AS PRESCRIBED BY THE PRIESTLY PHARMACIST *Xui*,' the other 'AS TOLD US BY A JEW FROM BYBLOS.' As well he provides against any obscure ailment of the eye not specifically dealt with by him:

REMEDY FOR THE EYE WHEN SOMETHING EVIL HAS HAPPENED TO IT

A Human Brain

Divide it in halves.

To one half add Honey and anoint the Eye therewith in the Evening.

Dry the other half, crush, powder, and anoint the Eye therewith in the Morning.

To correct Squint, Collyrium, Red-lead, and Soda were beaten into a paste and applied to the wandering eye. When the futility of this became apparent, a poultice of Onions, Granite, and Resin, was tried. This in turn failing to straighten the squinting optic, the animal world was combed for a remedy:

TO DRIVE AWAY SQUINTING IN THE EYES

Tortoise-brain	I
abra-ointment	I

Apply to the Eyes.

The final choice falling on the Tortoise because of the comparative rarity of cross-eyed tortoises in Ancient Egypt, it may be presumed.

Finally we have several remedies for 'Hotness in the Eyes,' a condition which without doubt must have been visited rather frequently on those driven for various reasons to place themselves under the care and treatment of an Oculist of the Pharaohonic period. As an eye-cooler 'Baked Ox-liver, placed carefully thereon' does not sound very hopeful, but Soda-from-Upper-Egypt (even when dissolved in Spring-water) sounds positively alarming in spite of the Scribe's special note appended to the prescription: 'IT HEALS IT!' The third remedy, however, shows more promise, and reveals once again a belief on the part of these ancient physicians in the homœopathic doctrine of like-curing-like:

ANOTHER TO DRIVE OUT HOTNESS IN THE EYES

Tallow-from-the-Jawbone-of-an-Ass

Mix in Cool Water and let the Patient put on his Temples in order that he may be healed forthwith.

CHAPTER XVII

DISEASES OF THE EAR, NOSE AND MOUTH

IN contradistinction to eye-troubles, affections of the Ears receive scant treatment. As might be expected, the chapter opens with a remedy for the Ear-that-Hears-Badly, but it is extremely doubtful if the sufferer experienced any relief from having his ears plugged with Red-lead and Resin-from-the-am-tree, even when rubbed up beforehand with Fresh Olive Oil.

For an Ear-that-Discharges-foul-smelling-Matter, an application of Incense-in-Goose-Grease ground up with Cream-from-the-Milk-of-a-Cow in various grains is recommended, but whether as poultice or injection is not altogether clear. Not that it mattered much, one is safe in asserting. Failing the above, an injection composed of Ass's Ear, Red-lead, Caraway and Olive Oil, could be squirted into the Ear. But discharging ears were as resistant to treatment in those days as in these, and detailed instructions were sometimes necessary:

ANOTHER TO TREAT THE EAR

Treat it with cooling remedies, not warm ones.

When the *met* trembles then make for him ut of Greenstone. Crush and apply for four days.

THEN MAKE HIM A CHARPIE:

Oil	$\frac{2}{3}$
Honey	the rest

Put frequently thereon.

When it flows out of his opening, then make him a ball which dries the wound:

Resin-of-Acanthus
Resin-of-the-Zizyphus-Lotus
Berry-of-the-Willow
Caraway

Crush and apply thereto.

When it is thick thereunder, MAKE FOR HIM THE REMEDY WHICH DRIES THE WOUNDS:

Head-of-the-amamu-animal
Gazelle's Ears
Tortoise-shell
annek-plant

Very frequently this stops it completely.

Make the same without delay. If it flows forth onto the earth, then it is a Healing-of-the-Ears; It clears up through the shooting-forth of the god Su. If it does not fall from him onto the earth, then make for him Slime-from-the-Greatness-of-that-which-presents-itself (i.e. the tumour), and enclose it in the Milky-Juice-of-the-Sycamore-Tree, that it may bind up his blood; neither Oil nor Honey put thereto;

cut off a half, as one would not wish that his Blood fall away from the other half . . . (uncertain). . . .

When afterwards thou recognizest that it has bound itself, so make thou for him:

Oil
Wax

Cook and plaster therewith.

Don't use too much.

Treat in the same way every swelling which breaks. If it goes off in abundance, then have a Linen band tied around the back of his head.

Considered in the light of more recent research it seems a pity for the sake of the patient that the Linen-band was not thought of in the first place and the remainder of the remedy conveniently forgotten.

Lastly, in the event of ulceration forming and extending into the Ear:

WHAT TO DO TO TREAT ULCERS WHICH EXTEND INTO THE EAR

There is a swelling internally. There is matter from the ulcers and from the dirt in his Ears, with fluid like Water-of-the-fermented-mes*x*a-drink. Go round the Ulcers with the Knife as far as there is Disease therein. Prepare for him Oil and Honey; put inside of it Charpie of Flax-of-a-cloth. Plaster it therewith so that it becomes well.

The nose is dealt with even more summarily than are the Ears, Coryza being the only condition mentioned. It could be treated by pouring Date-juice into the nostrils, or by rubbing the Nose with Peppermint-in-Dates; or much more vigorously, not to mention picturesquely, by a combination of Magic, Medicine and Surgery:

TO CHARM AWAY CORYZA

Spit it out, thou Slime, Son of Slime:
Grasp the bones, touch the skull, smear with tallow, give the patient seven openings in the head, serve the god Ra, thank the god Thoth.
Then I brought thy remedy for thee, thy drink for thee, to drive away, to heal it:
Milk-of-a-Woman-who-has-Borne-a-Son
Fragrant Bread
(Once again)
The Foulness rises from out the Earth!
The Foulness!
(Four times).

TO BE SPOKEN OVER THE MILK-OF-A-WOMAN-WHO-HAS-BORNE-A-SON AND FRAGRANT BREAD.
PUT IN THE NOSE.

Considering the indignities that we have seen put upon, or rather into, the mouth of the Ancient Egyptian by the physicians of the day, it is remarkable to note how lightly that cavity (with its contents) escaped serious damage. The diseased tongue is dismissed with a few simple remedies. At first a Milk-gargle is deemed sufficient:

BEGINNING OF THE REMEDIES TO DRIVE OUT DISEASES OF THE TONGUE

Milk

Gargle and put on the earth (i.e. spit out).

If the disease persisted, the Milk is reinforced by Goose-grease and the gargle turned into a chewing-remedy:

ANOTHER

amaa-grain
Goose-grease
Milk

Chew.

Another chewing-remedy was composed of Cow's Milk, Fresh Bread and Bullock's Fat; while still another could be prepared from Goose-Grease, Honey, Incense, Caraway-seeds, Fresh Lead-earth and Water, a specific instruction to chew it Nine Times being added.

As for the teeth, all that these appeared to need from time to time was 'strengthening,' which, after all, was not to be wondered at. Powdered-Fruit-of-the-Dom-palm with Honey effected this, we learn: it was rubbed on the teeth. If it did not, then Incense, Verdigris, and Fresh Lead-earth was tried; while extra-stubborn cases could try a still grittier preparation in the shape of Pebbles-powdered-in-Honey. The 'strengthening' process could also be carried out by the chewing method; Crocus-in-Sweet-Beer was one of the remedies recommended.

Gumboils (even the Ancients suffered from these painful afflictions!) were also found to yield to a chewing-remedy composed of Cow's Milk, Fresh Dates, and uah-grain, provided, however, it was kept moist and chewed Nine Times. And they also had 'Blisters-in-the-Teeth,' whatever they may mean. These were dealt with by a plaster which included Incense, Crocus, Cyperus, Onions, the Wood-of-Aloes, and Water, not to mention a variety of herbs of whose name and nature we are still in ignorance.

Chapter XVIII

THE NERVOUS SYSTEM

The proper interpretation to give to the word '*met*' has exercised the ingenuity of every Egyptologist who has essayed the translation of the various medical papyri which have survived to our day. Here, it undoubtedly refers to the nerves of the body; but there, it would appear just as undoubtedly to apply to the blood-vessels. Its exact interpretation then it is best to conclude rests on the state of knowledge enjoyed by these Ancients as to the anatomy of the human body: and that knowledge we can only gauge from papyri such as the one we are now concerned with.

If it were a mere matter of refreshing the *met*, a poultice of Fat-of-the-Ox, Fat-of-the-Ass, Fat-of-the-Ram, Fruit-of-the-Dompalm, *X*ehua-grain, Poppy-plant, and Sea-salt, served the purpose. To strengthen the *met* was likewise accomplished with no great amount of trouble, the choice of a variety of salves being given. One of these salves contained Cat's Oil; another Worm-oil; another had as an ingredient Leather-from-the-Sandal-maker! There was also a poultice:

ANOTHER TO STIMULATE AND TO STRENGTHEN THE *MET* IN EVERY LIMB

Flesh-of-a-Fat-Cow

Poultice the affected parts therewith.

To make the *met* supple was not so easy. One remedy advocated smearing the skin with a liniment composed of Bullock's fat, Yeast-of-Wine, Garlic, Saltpetre-from-the-South, Poppy-berries, and Oil-of-Myrrh. 'Do not let it dry' the Scribe added to the prescription; but apparently fearing that it would do so he hastened to add two further remedies for the 'dry parts of the *met*.' The first was surely an emergency remedy; it was a simple poultice of Cow's Milk and Beans. The second was more complicated, being a poultice of Watermelon, Fat-of-the-Egyptian-Goat, and Bullock's Flesh, seasoned with Garlic and Onions, and flavoured with Honey. Still more complicated and imposing was another poultice which boasted thirty-seven ingredients—the largest prescription in the Papyrus—and which numbered Hog's dung, Watermelon, and Goose-oil among those ingredients:

REMEDY TO MAKE THE *MET* SUPPLE

Fruit-of-the-Dompalm
Beans
amaa-grains
Onions

Splinters-of-the-Cedar-tree
Splinters-of-the-Mulberry-tree
Splinters-of-the-Willow-tree
Splinters-of-the-Zizyphus-Lotus
Splinters-of-the-Sycamore
Splinters-of-the-uan-tree
Resin-of-Acanthus
Resin-of-the-Zizyphus-Lotus
Resin-of-the-am-tree
Resin-of-the-Sycamore
Red-corn
Berries-of-the-am-tree
White Oil
Goose Oil
Hog's dung
Elderberries
Myrrh
Garlic
Herbs-of-the-Field
Thorns-of-the-Cyperus
Watermelon
Barley-plant
Fennel
abu-plant-from-the-Delta
Refuse-of-the-Flax-plant
Mineral-salt
anab-plant
Red-lead
Fresh-Lead-earth
Natron
Fat-of-the-Bullock

sasa-pieces

Make into one and poultice therewith.

For stubborn cases which defied the above remedies the ultimate resource was to a poultice composed of Human excrement macerated to a paste with Dates and Berries-of-the-Coriander.

On the whole the Scribe did this part of his work well. He prescribed remedies to strengthen the *met* of the Backbone, of the Shoulder, of the Thighs. 'For the *met* that runs to every limb' he recommended rubbing with a paste of Sour Milk and Breadcrumbs, warmed; while 'to protect the *met* in every limb' he counselled a poultice of Cow's Flesh, Cow's Bile, and Goat's Fat. 'For the *met* of the left side of the Body' he set down several remedies. One, an internal remedy, was compounded of Figs, Grapes, and Onions, Bread-of-the-Zizyphus-Lotus, Blossoms-of-the-Cucumber, Incense, Wine, and Sweet Beer. It was taken for four days. Irregularities of the *met* were cured by the patient chewing *uah*-grain while at the same time he clapped on to his buttocks a poultice of Goose's eggs—still another illustration of the Scribe's belief in the doctrine of like-curing-like.

As to the possibility of the human body assimilating the foregoing remedies there appears to have been a doubt in the mind of the Scribe. At any rate he very properly provided, or attempted to provide, against that eventuality, with what success it is not very difficult to estimate even at this distance of time:

REMEDY TO ALLOW THE *MET* TO TAKE UP THE REMEDY

Milk-of-a-Woman-who-has-borne-a-Son

Let it stand in a New Vessel until the Cream separates. Then smear the Patient.

Chapter XIX

THE ĀĀĀ DISEASE

Of all the difficulties that beset the translators of the Papyrus Ebers the most difficult centred around the diagnosis of the conditions which were continually cropping up in the text under the names of the ĀĀĀ disease, the u*x*edu-disease, and the uha-disease. Sometimes these conditions were described and treated separately. At other times they complicated each other sadly.

Three facts led at first to the ĀĀĀ disease being diagnosed as Bilharzia. These were firstly that throughout the papyrus the ĀĀĀ disease is almost invariably qualified by the adjective 'deadly.' Secondly the disease was specifically related to 'worms'; for example on Plate 19 of the Papyrus there appears a 'remedy to kill worms in the body that have been caused by the ĀĀĀ disease.' And thirdly that the symbol ĀĀĀ was always followed by a Phallus as the 'determinative sign.' This diagnosis of Bilharzia, however, is discarded by Joachim, who holds that the ĀĀĀ disease is in reality the common Egyptian scourge, Chlorosis Ægyptica, due to the intestinal parasite Ankylostomum duodenale, or Hookworm as it is more popularly known; and far from contradicting or belittling the three points set out above he turns them to his own advantage in support of his contention.

The first he disposes of by pointing out that the prefix 'deadly' was even more applicable to Chlorosis Ægyptica, for this scourge (according to the authority Griesinger) afflicted one out of every four of the population of Egypt. The second he waves aside on the ground that the 'worms' mentioned could apply equally to the Hookworm as to the Bilharzia parasite. Then as to the third point he insists that the use of the Phallus as the 'determinative sign' following the symbol ĀĀĀ must be viewed in the light of two other considerations: firstly that the Phallus is also the 'determinative sign' placed after ĀĀ, the symbol by which the much-mentioned Ass is designated in the Papyrus (a fact which very considerably diminishes the importance of its significance in the former case); and secondly that the use of the male generative organ in such a way is as easily applicable to Chlorosis Ægyptica as to Bilharzia since delayed puberty, impotence in males, and sterility in females, were frequent *sequelæ* of the Chlorosis.

As to the uha-disease and the uxedu-disease, Joachim holds that they are merely manifestations of the ĀĀĀ disease. The uxedu-disease, he declares, can be ascribed to the scourge in its early stages, although he is careful to point out that there are certain objections to that view which he cannot combat with satisfaction to himself. He feels on surer ground with the uha-disease, however, and unhesitatingly associates it with Chlorosis Ægyptica.

But whatever the diagnosis, and the balance of evidence is in favour of Joachim's contention, the multitudinous remedies proposed for the ĀĀĀ disease, whether by itself or complicated by the uha-disease or the u*x*edu-disease, brand it as a scourge of the first magnitude. Scores of 'remedies' are set down for combating its ravages, their number providing active proof (if such were needed) of the old adage that where there are many cures there is no cure. Added to which it can hardly be maintained that any one of the remedies proposed inspires a modern practitioner with any feeling of confidence in their success. To take a sample at random:

TO REMOVE THE ĀĀĀ-DISEASE

Jochauflegung of the sau-wood

Warm in Oil and give against it.

It may have been merely an oversight, though probably it was a wise precaution on the part of the Scribe, but whether the remedy was to be taken internally or externally is left in the extremest doubt.

For the uncomplicated u*x*edu the Scribe gives a series of mixtures to be taken, several ointments, and various suppositories. One mixture is in the nature of an infusion:

ANOTHER FOR THE u*X*EDU

Bark-of-the-Pomegranate-tree-soaked-in-Beer	$\frac{1}{3}$
Keep moist in a jug of Water	$\frac{5}{6}$

Strain a sufficient amount each morning and let the Patient drink.

There is no evidence that this remedy benefited the patient, but at least it could be drunk. This feat hardly seems possible with the next mixture in which the Flesh-of-a-Live-Cow was combined with Freshly-baked Bread, Incense, Lettuce, and Sweet Beer, and ordered to be ' drunk ' for four days. Another mixture of Ass's Milk with Dough, Wine, and Bitter Beer, was also ordered to be ' drunk ' for four days. All that one can say in its favour is that it appears on the surface to be somewhat more fluid than the other concoction.

Sometimes the u*x*edu caused spots to appear on the skin. A mixture of Onions, Turpentine, and Cow's Milk, drunk for four days, knocked the spots off. It would probably have the same effect if it were rubbed on.

When the u*x*edu-disease was complicated by the uha-disease the Scribe was rather at a loss. He counselled a salve of Sea-salt, Honey, and Cow's Bile; but at a later stage, having doubts as to the potency of Cow's Bile in this connection, he proceeded to repeat the salve, substituting however Cow's Brain for Cow's Bile. Even now he was not satisfied that the remedy would stand the test and seemingly in despair he resorted to what many a harried modern practitioner is driven to do to-day—he recommended a palliative. In this case it was the old familiar household remedy, Castor Oil, that he employed; but instead of administering it in the old familiar household way, namely a tablespoonful internally overnight, he ordered the oil to be rubbed in. Albeit, he took a roundabout way of saying so:

ANOTHER TO DRIVE OUT THE U*X*EDU

> Oil-expressed-from-the-Seeds-of-the-Castor-Oil-bush
>
> Smear therewith any person who has the uha-swelling with stinking matter. Lo, the Evil will be driven away as if nothing ailed him. Let him use the Oil in the same way for ten days as an Ointment, smearing himself twice in the early morning in order to drive away the disease as is proper.

But if the Scribe was at a loss before, he was certainly desperate when he came to deal with the 'wood-like uha-disease' occurring by itself. Salves were all that he could offer against it. They made up in picturesqueness what they most assuredly lacked in utility. An ointment of Hippopotamus Oil and Honey would perhaps be more sticky than picturesque. Another of Soot-from-the-bet'a-Pot with Honey and Sweet Myrrh would seem to be not only sticky but dirty. Another made of Ass's Head, Corn, and Oil, can only be called asinine, surely. A fourth, wherein

Stone-from-Memphis was ground up with Seeds and Grain in the Milk-of-a-Woman-who-has-borne-a-Son was without a doubt gritty. It had to be persisted in for seven days but does not seem to have been very successful since it was followed successively by other salves which had to be rubbed in for eight days, nine days, and ten days, respectively.

Finally there remained a salve calculated to arouse feelings of homicide in every poetic breast; a salve which sought to combine Seeds-from-the-Blossoms-of-the-Earth and Fresh Cream with the Hoof-of-an-Ass!

Chapter XX

THE HEART AND CIRCULATORY SYSTEM

To the student the most interesting section of the Papyrus is undoubtedly the chapter dealing with the Heart, or rather with the vascular system. At first sight one is in danger of assuming that the knowledge of the Heart and of its action enjoyed by these Ancients was much greater than it was in reality. But as one reads on it is clearly established that they made the fatal mistake of regarding the Heart not as a pump but as a mere well. Perhaps had they made a closer examination of the Heart itself they would have discovered the existence of the all-important valves, when (it is not too much to believe) they would in a flash have grasped the real function of the organ. For they had arrived at all save that. The section well merits setting down here at length. Unfortunately it cannot be set forth in its entirety for much of it is untranslatable, and indeed a great part of that which follows would seem to be sadly mistranslated; or so we must assume in all charity. But even allowing for this the Scribe reveals a knowledge of anatomy which is arresting, and the whole chapter calls for a revised translation which in the light of our present advanced knowledge of the language of the Ancients should definitely reveal how much real knowledge of the Heart and of the Blood Vessels they did possess.

THE BEGINNING OF THE SECRET BOOK OF THE PHYSICIAN

THE SCIENCE OF THE ACTION OF THE HEART AND OF THE HEART ITSELF

In the Heart are the vessels to the whole of the body. As to these every physician, every sexet-priest, every magician, will feel them when he lays his finger on the head, on the back of the head, on the hands, on the stomach (? heart) region, on the arms, on the legs. Everywhere he feels his Heart because its vessels run to all his limbs. Therefore it is called the centre of the vessels to all the limbs.

There are four vessels to the Nostrils, two of which convey mucus and two blood.

There are four vessels in the inside of either Temple. After they have given blood to the Eyes all kinds of diseases of the Eyes arise through them because they are open to the Eyes. When water comes out of them it is the Pupils of the Eyes that give it. Or according to another authority sleep in the Eyes brings it forth.

There arc four vessels which divide in the Head and spread out in the back thereof. These afterwards bring forth a great mass of hair. (Uncertain.)

When the breath goes into the Nose it makes its way to the Heart and Intestines, and the last-named vessels give to the body richly thereof. If one hears something below it is caused by the two vessels that go to the Collar-bone; or if one hears them thereunder, behold it is those that are in the upper Cheek-bones of a person in that it is the rough wind that cuts into him when he draws his breath therefrom. Or when the Heart absorbs Water his limbs fade away completely. When the Heart is struck it is that vessel whose name is 'Fasser' that does it; it gives water towards the Heart or towards the Eye when it is stopped up. When he hears through the opening of his mouth all his limbs show themselves benumbed after a mist has gripped his Heart. When anger arises in his Heart, behold it is a seething-up of the parts of the Intestine and the Liver. His Ear is on the alert, his vessels fall after their rising heat has dissolved everything.

There are four vessels to his Ears, two to the Right side and two to the Left. Breath-of-Life goes in the Right Ear and Breath-of-Death into the Left. Or in other words Breath-of-Life goes to the Right side and Breath-of-Death to the Left.

There are six vessels that run to the Arms, three to the Right and three to the Left, and they lead right down to the Fingers.

There are six vessels that lead to the Feet, three to the Right and three to the Left. They reach down to the Soles of the Feet.

There are two vessels to his Testicles which convey the Semen. There are two vessels to the Kidneys, one to one Kidney, the other to the second Kidney.

There are four vessels to the Liver which convey

to it Moisture and Air. Afterwards they cause all sorts of disease to arise therein being mixed with Blood.

There are four vessels to the Intestines and to the Spleen which likewise convey Moisture and Air. There are two vessels to the Bladder which convey the Urine.

There are four vessels which end in the Rectum. They give and bring forth in it Moisture and Air. Afterwards they turn towards the Rectum, each vessel to the Right and Left side right down to the Feet, mixing itself with the excrement.

When the Heart is sad, behold it is the moroseness of the Heart, or the vessels of the Heart are closed up in so far as they are not recognizable under thy hand. They grow full of Air and Water.

When the Heart feels an aversion, behold it is the Bitterness of the Heart because of Inflammation in the Anus. Thou findest it big and something forms itself in his Abdomen as in his Eye.

When his Heart spreads out, behold the vessels of the Heart are with excrement.

When any kind of dehert-disease enters the Left Eye and comes forth from the Navel, behold it is the Breath from the hollowed hand of the Priest that is allowed by the Heart to enter his vessels. Fire of every kind is locked up in his Flesh. His Heart is sick thereof because the Fire comes forth and the vessels of his Heart absolutely deny him their service.

When their clothes weigh them down, behold it is

the dehert-disease. When his dehert-disease breaks out, behold it is dangerous. (Uncertain.)

When the Heart is sick, behold there is an Oppression of the Heart, or it is an Overflow of Blood which arises in the Heart. It falls down and approaches his diaphragm, while his Heart feels an aversion.

When the mast-disease is in the Heart, behold there is a contraction of the Chest. His Heart has in its place Blood from the Anus which protrudes a little because of the disease. It is a Fever of the Heart. If his Heart quietens down a little under the disease he will eat, but only fastidiously.

When the Heart consumes itself, behold it is an Accumulation of Blood in the Heart. When there is mast-disease of the Heart because of the uxedu, behold his Heart is small in the inside of his Belly. The uxedu falls upon his Heart. He is aat-sick. He is mast-sick.

When there is Weakness as the result of old age, behold it is the uxedu at his Heart. When there is a rising of the Heart, behold it lifts itself at his left breast. It lifts itself on its fat. It flies forth from its place. Its layers of fat are on his Left Side so that they collect in his shoulder.

When the dehert-disease of his Heart appears frequently, behold his Heart swims and sinks downwards and is not in its place.

When his Heart is in its right place the Fat of the Heart is on the left side. It neither rises upwards nor falls downwards. It remains soundly in its place.

When his Heart trembles and there is much fat under his Left breast, behold it is his Heart which causes a little of the sinking because his disease is spreading.

When his Abdomen palpitates, it is caused by a swelling therein. When the Mouth is like Fire and becomes fatigued and the Heart is weary, behold it is because a Fire forces itself towards his Heart. His Heart burns with Fire like a person on whom fatigue has fallen.

When his heart experiences aversion like a person who has eaten the Bull-fruit of the Sycamore-tree, behold it is a veiling of his Heart like a person who has eaten the Bull-fruit of the Sycamore-tree.

When the Heart is miserable and is beside itself, behold it is the Breath of the heb-*x*er Priest that causes it through the hollow of his hand. It penetrates right down to the Rectum in such a manner that the Heart comes forth and loses its way under the disease.

When dryness befalls his Heart, behold it is the dryness of Fire that befalls it. He sighs often and his Heart is eaten up with anger; this is because his Heart is full of Blood, which in turn is due to drinking Warm Water and eating Bad Food.

When his Heart is afflicted and has tasted sadness, behold his Heart is closed in and darkness is in his body because of anger which is eating up his Heart.

When his Flesh is quite withered like the stilled Heart of a Person who has Found-the-Way (died), behold it is his Flesh which has become immovable under it, like the immovable flesh of a Person who has gone Into-the-Wide.

When it is Fate that he shall go Up-on-High, behold it is his Heart which determines that he shall go Up-on-High.

* * *

The section concludes with various remedies for affections of the heart, some of which are mixed up with a little 'anatomy':

Man has Twelve Heart-vessels which spread out to all his Limbs. There are Two Vessels in the region of his Breast which cause inflammation in the anus. Use against this:

Fresh Dates
Leaves-of-the-Castor-Oil-Plant
Fruit-of-the-Sycamore

Crush into one in Water, strain, and let it be taken for four days.

There are Two Vessels to his Thigh. When he suffers from his Thigh and both Thighs are a-tremble, say thou for it: 'This Vessel that runs to the region of his Thigh has conceived the disease.' Use against it:

Fresh Milk
Wormwood
Natron

Cook into one and make the Patient drink for four days.

There are Two Vessels to his Arm. When he suffers in his Arm and his fingers tremble, then thou sayest to him: 'They are swollen glands.' Prepare against them: Fish-glue in Beer, and t'as-plant or Flesh in Watermelon, and poultice his fingers. Thereby he will become well.

When he is ill in his neck and has pains in both eyes, then say to him: 'It is the vessels of the neck which have taken up the disease.' Prepare against it:

Sap-of-the-*X*et'-tree
A Farmer's Urine
Elderberry
Berry-of-the-sames-plant
Mix in Honey and poultice his neck therewith for four days.

There are Two Vessels in his Occiput, Two to his Forehead, Two to his Eyes, Two to his Eyebrow, Two to his Nostril, Two to his Right Ear and Breath-of-Life goes through them, Two to his Left Ear and Breath-of-Death goes through these. They come entirely from his Heart and divide themselves in his Nose, collecting themselves entirely in his Back-cheeks. The diseases of the anus are carried off by them by their outflow. They are brought hither by the Thigh-vessels from the Beginning until Death.

Numerous other remedies for the Heart find place here and there in other parts of the Papyrus. To drive out disease in the Heart one remedy of Milk, Honey, and Water, had simplicity if nothing else to commend it. If it did not act one proceeded automatically to a stronger mixture of Onions, Sweet Beer and Date-meal. For Fever-in-the-Heart the Blossoms-of-the-Cucumber were urged; or the Cucumber itself, mashed up into a 'drink' with Honey, Dates, Dough, and Water, could be used. Then, to leave no loop-hole, a remedy to heal the heart 'for certain' was given: Figs one-eighth part, Fresh Lead-earth one-sixteenth, Cake one-thirty-second, and Water five-sixths was said to encompass this end.

In addition one finds a dozen remedies to 'put the Heart into proper working order and make it take up nourishment.' Like many another remedy in the Papyrus they do not on the face of them appear very promising, although very little exception can be taken to the simpler ones such as Corn and Sweet Beer, or Wine and Grain-of-Wheat, especially since they were to be taken for one day only. But most of the other remedies were tougher propositions, for tough is the only designation applicable to a 'drink' which is composed of Fat Flesh, Figs, Berries, Incense, Caraway, Nasturtium, Goose-grease, Writing-fluid, and Sweet Beer; or to a concoction of Fat Flesh, Figs, Dates, Incense, Garlic, and Sweet Beer—with Willow-tree, one-eighth part, added as a stiffening.

Chapter XXI

DIAGNOSIS

The efforts at diagnosis, samples of which are given hereunder, reveal a commendable amount of observation on the part of the ancient physician, quaintly expressed though the results of that observation be. But though they be quaintly expressed, which of us could improve on that phraseology? The mental picture that is conjured up by the description of the patient who was ' not in a condition to jump the Nile,' or of that other patient whose abdomen was ' as weak as a woman who has had a child '; or of the tumour that ' goes and comes under the fingers like oil-in-a-tube,' or of that other tumour whose ' point is high-uplifted like a woman's breast,' is as complete as any modern diagnostician could paint it.

Whilst most of the growths dealt with hereunder are handed over to the physician for treatment, the surgeon is not absolutely ignored. About a dozen cases in all fall to him. In some he is directed to use the Cautery, in others the Knife—being admonished to beware of the vessels in so doing. In one case he is directed to first use the Knife and then to check the Hæmorrhage by means of the Cautery. In only one condition in the whole Papyrus is a policy of masterly inactivity advocated: this is in the case of a tumour of the god *X*ensu. 'Do thou nothing there against!' is the warning the Scribe gives after describing this 'loathsome disease,' as he labels it.

*   *   *

When thou Examinest a Person who suffers from an Obstruction in his Abdomen and thou findest that it goes-and-comes under thy fingers like oil-in-a-tube, then say thou: 'It all comes from his mouth like slime!' Prepare for him:

Fruit-of-the-Dompalm
Dissolve in Man's Semen
Crush, cook in Oil and Honey

To be eaten by the Patient for four mornings. Afterwards let him be smeared with dried, crushed, and pressed maqut-grain.

*   *   *

When thou Examinest a Person who suffers from an Obstruction in his Abdomen and he feels discomfort after he has taken food, his body swells up, his heart is weak; when he walks it is like a person who is suffering from an inflammation in his Anus: let him lie outstretched and examine him. If thou findest that his body is hot and his abdomen hard, then say thou to him: 'This is a Liver complaint.' Make for him the Secret Remedy that the Physician has prescribed:

pa*x*estet-plant
Refuse-of-dates

Mix, dissolve in Water, and let the Patient drink for four mornings so that thou wilt empty his body.

When thou findest, after this has come to pass, the Right side of his body hot, and the Left side cool, then say thou: 'This illness is in process of healing. It is consuming itself.' SEE HIM AGAIN. If thou findest that his body has cooled down then thou sayest: 'His Liver has healed and cleansed itself. He has absorbed the medicine.'

* * *

WHEN THOU EXAMINEST THE OBSTRUCTION IN HIS ABDOMEN and thou findest that he is not in a condition to leap the Nile, his stomach is swollen and his chest asthmatic, then say thou to him: 'It is the Blood that has got itself fixed and does not circulate.' Do thou cause an emptying by means of a medicinal remedy. Make him therefor:

Wormwood	$\frac{1}{8}$
Elderberries	$\frac{1}{16}$
sebesten	$\frac{1}{8}$
sasa-chips	$\frac{1}{8}$

Cook in Beer-that-has-been-brewed-from-many-ingredients, strain into one, thoroughly, and let the Patient drink.

This remedy drives out blood through his mouth or rectum which resembles Hog's Blood when-it-is-cooked. Either make him a poultice to cool him in front, or thou dost not prepare him this remedy, but makest for him the following really excellent Ointment composed of:

Ox fat
Saffron seeds
Coriander
Myrrh
aager-tree

Crush and apply as a poultice.

* * *

WHEN THOU EXAMINEST A PERSON WHO HAS A HARDENING, his stomach hurts him, his face is pale, his heart thumps; when thou examinest him and findest his heart and stomach burning and his body swollen, then it is the sexen-illness in the Depths and the fire is consuming him. Make him a remedy that quenches the fire and empties his bowels by drinking Sweet-Beer-that-has-stood-in-dry-Dough. This to be eaten and drunk for Four days. Look every morning for six days following at what falls from his rectum. If excrement fall out of him like little black lumps, then say to him: 'The body-fire has fallen from the stomach. The asi-disease in the body has diminished.' If thou examinest him after this has come to pass and something steps forth from his rectum like the white of beans and drops shoot forth out of him like nesu-of-tepaut, then thou sayest: 'What was in his abdomen has fallen down.' MAKE FOR HIM THIS REMEDY SO THAT HIS FACE MAY COOL. Stand the cauldron over the fire, make a mixture in it and cook it in the usual way.

To drive away the Hardening in the Abdomen:

Bread-of-the-Zizyphus-Lotus	1
Watermelon	1
Cat's dung	1
Sweet Beer	1
Wine	1

Make into one and apply as a poultice.

* * *

When thou Examinest a Person with a Hardening in his Abdomen, his stomach hurts him, discomfort seizes him after every meal, his abdomen is swollen, he suffers in both his feet, the soles of his feet, but not in his ankles; if thou examinest him and find his abdomen as weak as a woman-who-has-had-a-child, and his head is weak, then say thou to him: 'It is a stoppage of excrement.' Water penetrates into him as if it had hopped in . . . (uncertain). . . . Make for him the remedy from the Secret Book that is only for the Physician with the exception of thine own daughter:

Green undried Wheat

Cool in Water without evaporating it. Take it off the Fire in order to mix Refuse-of-Dates with it. Strain and let him take it for four days so that he may be immediately cured.

* * *

When thou Examinest a Person with a Hardness in his Left side, he has feet that he-cannot-walk-with, then say thou: 'He has dug sand-bags and lifted sand.' Prepare for him the remedy that is mentioned before:

Fruit-of-the-Dompalm	$\frac{1}{4}$
am-seeds, crushed	$\frac{1}{2}$
Elderberries	$\frac{1}{16}$
sasa-chips	$\frac{1}{8}$

Cook into one with Oil, one, and Honey, a little, and let the Patient eat for Four days.

* * *

When thou Examinest a Person who is ill in his Abdomen, all his limbs are heavy like a person who goes-to-lie-down, lay thy hand on his abdomen. If thou findest that his abdomen is swollen and that it comes-and-goes under thy fingers, they say thou: 'The fault lies in the digestion of his food.' At first do not let him eat. Prepare a radical purge for him:

Refuse-of-Beer

Dissolve in Flat Beer.

Afterwards let him go and eat his bread. If thou examinest him after this has come to pass and thou findest the small of his back warm and his body cool, then say thou: 'The fault in the emptying of the bowels has cleared up.' Let him guard his mouth against everything hot.

* * *

When thou Examinest any Person who is suffering in his Abdomen, and thou findest after he has leapt the Nile that he is ill in both sides, his body is swollen, when he takes nourishment his stomach feels uncomfortable at its entrance, then it is the be*x*etu-illness. Fight thou against it with soothing-remedies after he has had a poultice of Wheat-water. If it moves hereafter under thy fingers then give him an enema for four mornings. Their injection is painful. Against this use

uah-grain	$\frac{1}{2}$
Gum-drops	$\frac{1}{8}$
Fresh lead-earth	$\frac{1}{16}$

Cook in Oil and Honey and let the patient take for four days.

If it afterwards moves under thy fingers like grains of sand, and all his limbs burn with the itch—

Fermenting Bread
Some Horn
Duck's Food

goes into him as if it hopped in . . . (uncertain). . . .

* * *

When thou Examinest a Person with a suffering in his Abdomen, he is ill in his arm, in his breasts, and in the stomach-region; and it is told him that it is the uat-illness (literally the green, blooming, and fresh illness), then thou sayest: 'It is Death that has penetrated his mouth and taken up its abode.' Make him a stinging remedy from the following plants:

tehua-berry	1
Poppy-plant	1
Peppermint	1
annek-plant	1
Red-se*x*et-seeds	1

Cook in Oil and let the Patient drink.

LAY THOU THY HAND ON HIM. HIS ARM IS EXTENDED WITH EASE, FREE FROM PAIN. THEN SAY THOU: 'This suffering has passed the real intestinal passage to the rectum. I will not repeat the medicine.'

* * *

WHEN THOU EXAMINEST A PERSON WHO IS SUFFERING IN HIS ABDOMEN, it breaks often and thou findest something like a projection on his ventral side; both his eyes are tired and his nose stopped up. Then say thou: 'It is a fault in his excrement. It does not pass through his intestines as waste matter.' Make him for it:

Wheaten-bread
Wormwood-in-particularly-large-quantities

Thereto add a small vessel with Garlic along with broken pieces of the same with Beer and Fat Flesh-from-an-Ox. Let the Patient eat and drink this with Beer-that-has-been-brewed-from-many-ingredients in order to open his eyes, to open his nose, and to make easy the passing of his excrement.

* * *

WHEN THOU EXAMINEST A PERSON WHO IS SUFFERING IN HIS ABDOMEN, his limbs are tender and quite flaccid; thou examinest him and findest no wound on his body except in the genitals . . . (uncertain) . . . like a little ball, then say thou to him: 'There is something dangerous in thee.' Make him as a remedy against it:

Hæmatite-from-Elefantine, crushed
Linseed
Onions
Cook in Oil and Honey.

Let the Patient eat this for four mornings in order to quench his thirst and to drive away the dangerous matter from his stomach.

* * *

When thou Examinest a Person who is suffering in his Abdomen and findest something in his backbone like the trouble in the knife-grinder's disease, then thou sayest: 'This is the uxedu that has spread to his back. He is ill. I will make him the Back-remedy. It goes into him as if it had hopped in. Make for him a pot-yeast and then make him the following remedy:

Spring Plant	1
Peppermint	1
Resin-of-Acanthus	1
Mason's Clay	1

Crush, cook in Yeast-of-Sweet-Beer, and smear on for four days in order to heal him at once.

* * *

When thou Examinest a Person who from time to time has Pains like those who have

EATEN UNCLEAN THINGS, his heart is feeble as if the frailty of old age has overcome him . . . (uncertain) . . . then say thou: 'It is an accumulation of morbid juices.' He shall not wilfully minimize the danger nor put his trust in feeble remedies. An abscess has formed. There is putrid matter in it and a discharge from the wound. Make him the remedy for opening it. (The prescription, however, was overlooked!)

* * *

WHEN THOU MEETEST A GROWTH IN THE NECK OF A PERSON WHICH HAS ARISEN IN CONJUNCTION WITH IRRITATION OF THE ATUT IN ANY PART OF THE BODY OF A PERSON WHEREIN THERE IS MATTER, and thou findest its point high-uplifted like a woman's breast, and the matter moves therein, then say thou: 'He has a growth in his neck in which the matter moves. I will treat the illness.' Prepare against it the following healing remedy:

Garlic
Palm-juice
*X*ehui-grains
Caraway
Sea-salt
Yeast
Bean-meal
Berry-of-the-sames-plant
Honey
aber-oil

Mix into one and poultice therewith for four days so that he may become well.

* * *

WHEN THOU MEETEST A GROWTH IN THE NECK OF A PERSON WITH AN IRRITATION OF THE ATUT WHICH IS IN FRONT, and thou findest it as though it were a cover thereon; it is soft under thy fingers and there is something there like corn, then thou sayest: 'He has a growth of fat with an irritation of the atut in his neck. I WILL TREAT THE ILLNESS.' Make thou the remedy against it which will cause its disappearance by soothing means:

Saltpetre
teun-plant
Wasp's Blood
Ox Bile
Sea-salt
Bean-meal

Crush and poultice therewith for four days.

* * *

WHEN THOU MEETEST A GROWTH OF THE ATUT WHICH HAS LASTED FOR MANY DAYS, there is dirt in it, it forms a fatty swelling and the greater part of it is hot, then say thou: 'He has a growth of the atut that has caused an accumulation of matter. Dirt has formed in it and it is hot underneath. I will fight the disease.' Prepare against it the remedy that heals it, that drives it away by means of the following:

Dried Blood
Caraway
Oil
Onions
Resin-of-Acanthus
Fruit-and-Nut-of-Acanthus
Seezunge-grains
Copper Coal

Make into a Pill.

* * *

When thou meetest a Fatty Growth in the Neck and findest it like an Abscess of the Flesh that is soft under thy finger . . . (gap in the text) . . . then say thou: ' He has a fatty growth in his neck. I will treat the disease with the Knife, taking care of the Blood-vessels the while.' Prepare against it a poultice as a healing remedy which frees the pustules:

teun-plant
*X*ehui-plant
Berry-of-the-sames-plant
Blood-of-the-nehur-bird
Wasp's Blood
sasa-chips
amamu-plant
Lead-vitriol
Sea-salt

Crush, make into one, and poultice therewith.

* * *

When thou meetest a Mattery-Tumour in the Neck of a Grown-up Man, it forms an elevation, brings forth fleshy masses of matter and lasts years or months; matter comes forth therefrom like fluid from a Stickleback-fish or the Great Scorpion, then say thou: 'He has a mattery-tumour. I will fight the disease.' Prepare against it the remedy to draw the pustules out of his neck:

Wax
Cow's fat
*X*et-plant
Writing-fluid
teun-plant
Caraway
Copper-shavings
Verdigris
Fresh lead-earth
Sea-salt
Goose-fat
Incense-berries
Collyrium

Cook and poultice the neck therewith.

* * *

When thou meetest a Tumour of the Flesh in any part of the Body of a Person, and thou findest it like hide in his flesh; he is clammy; it goes-and-comes under thy finger except when the finger is kept still because the matter escapes through it, then thou sayest: 'It is a Tumour of the

Flesh. I will treat the disease. I will try to heal it with Fire like the Cautery heals.'

* * *

WHEN THOU MEETEST A TUMOUR THAT HAS ATTACKED A VESSEL, it has formed a tumour in his body when thy finger examines it, and it is hard like a hard stone under thy fingers, then say thou: 'It is a Tumour of the Vessels. I will treat the disease with the Knife.' Poultice it with Fat. Treat it as one would treat a suppurating wound in any part of the body of a person.

* * *

WHEN THOU MEETEST A FAT TUMOUR IN ANY PART OF THE BODY OF A PERSON and thou findest that it comes-and-goes under thy fingers while it also trembles when thy hand stands still, then say thou: 'It is a Fat Tumour. I will treat the disease.' Treat it with the Knife as one heals an open wound.

* * *

WHEN THOU MEETEST A TUMOUR OF THE U*x*EDU IN THE HEAD . . . (uncertain) . . . and thou findest that it produces fluid, that it grows under thy fingers when they are kept still, and that it is soft even if it is not large, then say thou: 'It is a tumour of the u*x*edu in the Head . . . (uncertain). . . . I will treat the disease. Treat it with the Knife but contrive that thou avoidest the blood-vessels. Something flows thereout like Cake-water. There is a shaggy covering fastened thereto. Let nothing thereof remain behind, let nothing run about. Heal it as one heals an open wound in any part of the body of a person, and heal the vessels. The pustules that a person gets, let them swell up and drive them away afterwards . . . (uncertain). . . .

* * *

When thou meetest a Growth that has arisen in conjunction with the Irritation of the U*x*edu and thou findest it like beans, discharging abscesses arise in his skin, not large it is true; when the person is ill with pus in the inside of his body, then say thou to him: 'He has a growth of the u*x*edu which has developed pus. I will treat the disease.' Make thou against it the remedy which frees the pustules and drives out the matter:

teun-plant
*X*ehui-berries
Wasp's Blood
Sea-salt
Watermelon
hemit-grains
Powdered amaa-plant
Bean-meal
Bullock's fat
Wax

Cook and poultice therewith in order that he may become well.

* * *

When thou meetest a Tumour of the Vessels in any part of the Body of a Person and thou findest it round in form, growing under thy finger, and spread out against the flesh; it is not big and does not protrude; then say thou: 'It is a tumour of the *met*. I will treat the disease. The *metu* causes it and it then becomes a pricking of the *met*.' Treat it with the Knife and burn it with Fire so that it bleeds not too much. Heal it like the Cautery heals.

* * *

When thou meetest a Tumour of the Metu on the inner side of any Limb, it grows and thou seest that it winds itself like snakes while it forms many prominences and these are like things that are moved by the wind, then say thou: 'It is a tumour of the *metu*.' Do not knock it with a knock again because this pricks the limb through its knocking. Prepare and take care of the *metu* in every part of the limb of a person. (Here follows a Magic Formula which is to be repeated for four mornings. It is incomprehensible to us and impossible of translation.)

* * *

When thou meetest a large Tumour of the god *Xensu* in any part of the Limb of a Person, it is loathsome and suffers many pustules to come forth; something arises therein as though wind were in it, causing irritation. The Tumour calls with a loud voice to thee: " Is it not like the most loathsome of pustules?' It mottles the skin and makes figures. All the limbs are like those which are affected. Then say thou: '*It is a Tumour of the god Xensu. Do thou nothing there against.*'

* * *

When thou meetest a Skin-Tumour on the outside part of the Body above his Genitals, lay thy finger on it and examine his body, palpating with thy fingers. If his bowels move and he vomits at the same time, then say thou: 'It is a Skin-Tumour in his body. I will treat the disease by heat to the bladder on the front of his body which causes the tumour to fall to the earth.' When it is so fallen, then make thou for him warm so that it may pierce his body . . . (uncertain). . . . Heal it as the Cautery heals.'

* * *

When thou meetest a Pustular Tumour in the limb of a Person and if on palpating it thou findest that it goes-and-comes and that the flesh that is thereunder is drawn over, then say thou: 'A gathering of Pustules!' Use the Knife against it. Bore through it with the Knife. Work with the hennu-animal. Work what is on the inner side with the hennu-animal. Cut it with the Knife.

There is Largeness therein. There is something therein like the *menter* of the mouse. Cut it loose. Lead forth these *aderu* that are on his side. Cover the body with cuts. Work it with one hennu-vessel of Onions . . . (uncertain). . . .

Chapter XXII

THE HAIR

The man has yet to be born who will not be thrilled on learning that the very first remedy for Baldness recorded in history was prepared for a woman—and for a Queen at that! Composed of

Toes-of-a-Dog
Refuse-of-Dates
Hoof-of-an-Ass

it was compounded nearly five thousand years ago as a Remedy for Hair-Growth prepared for Ses, Mother of His Majesty the King of Upper and Lower Egypt, Teta, deceased.

The chapter on the hair is throughout an illuminating one. It reveals the fact that fifty centuries ago the human race was wrestling just as feverishly as now with the twin problems of grey hair and baldness. A first glance at the extraordinary concoctions recommended in this special chapter to check the effects of age on the hair fill the reader with disgust. Further consideration of the chapter, however, tones down that feeling to some extent. It is very evident that in this section of the Papyrus the Scribe was simply copying from other sources, for he has observed no order whatever in the entries but simply dashed down the remedies as they came to him. If they be re-arranged one can say this much for these pioneer cosmetic-physicians that at least in the first place they were content with simply recommending oil without any admixture to stimulate the growth of the hair; and it was only after age or disease had won through, and grey locks and bald patches showed themselves, that they resorted to desperate remedies.

Already in a previous chapter we have been presented by the Scribe with a short but pithy dissertation on the virtues and uses of Castor Oil, and we have seen that God-given drug especially recommended to women for increasing the growth of the hair. Another hair-restorer that has a familiar ring about it consists of Linseed crushed in Oil and rubbed on the head. Still another simple remedy was one which seems to contain in it the first germ of the hair-brush idea:

ANOTHER TO CAUSE THE HAIR TO GROW

Hair-of-the-hunta-animal

Warm in Oil and rub the Head therewith for four days.

However, simple remedies having failed to stem the tide of years as reflected in the colour or the scarcity of the hair, the plunge is taken and an array of remedies suggested, the very mention of which is almost sufficient to activate the hair-cells out of sheer terror. Some are merely quaint, as for example the Tooth-of-an-Ass mixed in Honey and rubbed on the scalp; or highly inconvenient such as a lotion of Writing-fluid and Brain-water, for falling hair; or mighty bewildering, as witness:

ANOTHER FOR THE GROWTH OF THE HAIR ON A HEAD WHICH IS BECOMING BALD

Fat-of-the-Lion
Fat-of-the-Hippopotamus
Fat-of-the-Crocodile
Fat-of-the-Cat
Fat-of-the-Serpent
Fat-of-the-Egyptian-Goat

Make into one and rub the head of the Bald One therewith.

But other preservatives and restoratives are frankly and positively revolting, such as a concoction of Writing-fluid, Fat-of-the-Hippopotamus, and Gazelle's dung; and another which is a vile concoction of Vulva, Phallus, and the Black Lizard—plus some other ingredients which (perhaps fortunately) cannot be deciphered. Not quite so revolting are the several remedies which aim at once at preserving the hair and removing grey hairs. The Blood-of-a-Black-Calf, cooked in Oil, figures in one such; the same of a Black Cow in another; while a third is composed of Tortoise-shell and the Neck-of-the-gabgu-bird, cooked in Oil.

Whether these Ancient Egyptians were in any way

cognisant of the selective action of the Thyroid Gland on the hair, or whether indeed the gabgu-bird possessed a Thyroid at all, the fact remains that they must have imagined they had found some specific for hair-growth in the neck of this unknown bird; for in another prescription we find 'Blood-from-the-Neck-of-the-gabgu-bird' not only recommended, but backed up by a word-picture of the fortunate user which appears to be nothing less than the first attempt on earth to describe 'that Kruschen feeling," so much advertised:

ANOTHER REMEDY TO PREVENT GREY HAIRS

Blood-from-the-Neck-of-the-gabgu-bird

Put in Real Balsam and rub therewith.

HE STRETCHES UP HIS HAND TO THE BACK OF A LIVING FALCON, PLACING HIM ON HIS HEAD AGAINST A LIVING SWALLOW!

Almost it reads like the daily paper account of the after-results of a gland-graft, but actually it is understood that the Scribe merely wishes to convey that the medicament overcomes the disease like the Falcon the Swallow.

The remedies for dyeing grey hairs provide powerful sermons on the vanity of old or of middle-old age. Rubbing the head with the Horn-of-a-Fawn, warmed in Oil, was recommended. As a hair-dye it leaves much to be desired, but for all that it had its points and was infinitely to be preferred to the remaining remedies. For the 'Bile-of-Many-Crabs' conjures up a messy mass, and a smelly one too; and 'Dried-Tadpoles-from-the-Canal, crushed in Oil' does not sound much better. Both of course were applied to the outside of the head. They are mild, however, compared to two others: one, the Womb-of-a-Cat warmed in Oil with the Egg-of-the-gabgu-bird, and rubbed into the cropped head; the other, Hoof-of-an-Ass, roasted, Vulva-of-a-Bitch, a Black Tapeworm, and the uauit-worm-which-is-found-in-dung: the whole cooked in Oil and Gum and rubbed well into the scalp! Grey eye-brows, let it be said hurriedly, were not so obstinate as the grey hairs of the head; if they did not yield to an application of Crocodile-earth-mixed-with-Honey-which-has-been-dissolved-in-Onion-water, one could still try Ass's Liver warmed in Oil with Opium. This latter remedy was to be made up into little balls with which one rubbed the grey eye-brows.

Alopecia (that is the unsightly bald patches which appear suddenly on the heads of people old and young, male and female) may be noted here although it is treated elsewhere in the Papyrus. It could be attacked in three ways. Quills-of-the-Porcupine could be warmed in Oil and used against it; or Red-lead beaten up in Froth-of-Bitter-Beer. Both were external remedies, one presumes. A third method lay in shaving the head and applying to it a Broken-up-Figure-warmed-in-Oil-which-has-been-mixed-with-Writing-fluid-in-Water. Or just as suitable as any of these was Flax-plant-mixed-in-Oil-with-Wasp's-dung. Still another method was if anything more interesting since it invoked the Sun's rays:

TO CHARM AWAY ALOPECIA

O Shining One, Thou who hoverest above!
O *X*are! O Disc of the Sun!
O Protector of the Divine Neb-apt!

To be spoken over

Iron
Red-lead
Onions
Alabaster
Honey

Make into one and give against.

Wonderful to relate this remedy after all these centuries still persists. For it is still the Sun's rays (in the shape of Artificial Sunlight) that we invoke for Alopecia; and we still retain the Iron Tonic of the Ancients, although we have long discarded the Red-lead, Onions, Alabaster, and Honey, as of doubtful benefit.

Not the least interesting entries in this chapter on the hair are the three prescriptions which bring it to a close. One, to remove superfluous hairs, recommends the frequent rubbing in of a mixture compounded of Tortoise-shell crushed and heated in Fat-from-the-Hoof-of-a-Hippopotamus: probably on the theory that superfluous hairs are seldom, if ever, found on the shell of the Tortoise nor on the hoof of the Hippopotamus. The other two prescriptions remind us even more sharply of the unchangeableness of human nature despite all the water that has flowed between the banks of the Nile since they were written down. They are also to remove hair, but in each case the oily mass is curtly directed 'TO BE POURED OVER THE HEAD OF THE HATED WOMAN.' It would appear from this peep into the past that it was only at a later stage of our civilization that hair-pulling became a female accomplishment.

Chapter XXIII

COSMETICS

Next to losing her hair the greatest terror of a woman's life is the wrinkle (or rather, wrinkles, since they never come singly) and it would seem that their appearance was resented thousands of years ago just as fiercely as in this twentieth century. Let us see how the Ancients dealt with them:

TO DRIVE AWAY WRINKLES FROM THE FEATURES

Incense-cake
Wax
Fresh Olive Oil
Cyperus

Crush, grind, put in Fresh Milk, and apply to the face for six days.

See to it!

We need have no doubt but that the ladies of the day 'saw to it!' But wrinkles are not the only things that mar a woman's peace of mind; a spotty or a blotchy complexion is just as great a disturber of sleep, and in the search for that school-girl complexion some of the methods used by the Ancient Egyptiennes were not so far removed from those employed by her modern sister:

TO MAKE THE FACE SMOOTH

Cake-meal in Well-water

After she has washed her face daily, let her anoint her face with it.

But if there are some of the moderns who pin their faith to Milk in order to preserve their complexions at least it is of the bovine brand:

ANOTHER REMEDY

Water-from-the-qebu-plant
Meal-of-Alabaster
Fresh abt-grain

Mix in Honey, make into a pap, mix in Human Milk, and anoint the face therewith.

The next remedy was surely reserved for those from whom the second and third, as well as the first bloom of youth had departed:

ANOTHER REMEDY

Bullock's Bile
Whipped-up Ostrich Egg
Oil
Dough
Refined Natron
Hautet-resin

Mix, make into a pap, mix in Fresh Milk, and wash the face therewith daily.

To remove a mole nothing was left to chance and internal and external medications were made use of:

REMEDY AGAINST A MOLE

Berries-of-the-t'as-plant
mamer-grain
Pound, and let the person take who has the Mole.
Honey
Leaf-of-the-mamer-corn

Crush in Water-with-which-the-Phallus-has-been-Washed: therewith plaster it one night that it may remain on his arms and his limbs.

It was a simple matter to alter the colour of the skin; not even a trip to the sea-side was necessary. Instead, some Sea-salt could be brought to one's abode, there rubbed up with Honey and Red Natron, and the colour of the skin altered by anointing the body with the sticky mixture. Another sticky mass was said to beautify the body:

REMEDY TO BEAUTIFY THE SKIN

Meal-of-Alabaster
Meal-of-Natron
Sea-salt
Honey

Mix into one in this Honey and anoint the body therewith.

Finally—with a thoroughness that does them credit—we find the cosmetic preparations supplemented by a remedy for Sweaty Feet:

REMEDY TO DRIVE AWAY SWEATY FEET IN A PERSON

uadu-plant-of-the-Fields
Eel-from-the-Canal
Warm in Oil and smear both feet therewith.

Chapter XXIV

DOMESTIC HINTS

Strictly speaking this chapter should be headed Domestic and Farmyard Hints, for it comprehends the barn as well as the cradle, rats and scorpions in addition to fleas and lice. To begin with the cradle:

REMEDY TO STOP THE CRYING OF A CHILD

> Pods-of-the-Poppy-plant (Opium)
> Fly-dirt-which-is-on-the-Wall
>
> Make into one, strain, and take for four days.
> It acts at once!

This is startling! No other word can convey the amazement with which one finds that the means employed to quell the squalling infant five thousand years ago are identically the same as many a modern mother employs to-day. Let us compare them:

REMEDY TO STOP THE CRYING OF A CHILD
(NEW STYLE)

> Powder-which-contains-Opium
> Fly-dirt-which-is-on-the-Dummy

Mix in the Child's mouth.
IT ACTS AT ONCE!

Only slightly less startling is another recipe from out that far-distant past:

TO KEEP MICE AWAY FROM CLOTHES

Cat's Fat

Smear on everything possible.

Nowadays our expansive wardrobes, not to mention other prejudices, prohibit this method, but it is still the cat which we employ to keep the mice away.

It is rather more difficult to trace any resemblance between ancient and modern customs in the remaining recipes in this chapter. Our custom of swathing the whole body in close-fitting garments is, perhaps, responsible for this in certain cases as, for example, in the following:

BEGINNING OF THE REMEDIES TO DRIVE AWAY FLEAS AND MICE

Date-meal
Water

Cook to one portion in two hennu-vessels and drink warm. Afterwards let him spit it out in order to drive away the Fleas and Lice that desport themselves on his limbs.

It is only natural to expect that a people who took such active steps to prevent objectionable vermin like fleas and lice from ‘ desporting themselves on their limbs ’ should exhibit a laudable desire to sweeten their homes and their persons. As will be seen they went further and bestowed attention on their breath:

SUBSTANCES TO USE IN ORDER TO MAKE PLEASANT THE SMELL OF THE HOUSE OR OF THE CLOTHES

Dried Myrrh
Elderberries
Incense
Cyperus
Resin-of-Aloes
sebet-resin
Calmus-from-the-land-t'ahi-in-Asia
inekuun-grain
mastich
styrax

Crush, grind, make into one, and put on the fire.

ANOTHER FOR THE WOMAN TO MAKE THEREOUT

These ingredients, according to the other instructions, put in Honey, cook, mix, form into little balls. They shall fumigate with them. It is also worth while to make Mouth-pills out of them to make the smell of the mouth agreeable.

Having dispersed the fleas and lice from their

limbs, sweetened their homes, their clothes, their breath, and their feet, removed wrinkles and moles from their faces and restored the softness of youth to their cheeks, it can be understood that they were not going to allow vermin to overrun their homes. Consequently we find several remedies directed to that end:

TO DRIVE VERMIN OUT OF THE HOUSE

Do thou sprinkle it with Natron-Water. By that means they are dispersed.

ANOTHER

bebet-plant

Crush in Oil and carefully sprinkle the house therewith. Thereby they are dispersed.

The Farmyard in Egypt must have been an interesting place. We are told what to do to prevent Wasps stinging: we simply take the Fat-of-the-bird-coracias-garrula and smear ourselves with it. To prevent the Tarantula stinging, however, inunction with Olive Oil was sufficient. If a Scorpion got in our way, we immediately seized a Lizard and put it on the fire. The Scorpion died. If, however, we met a Lizard—they must have been more ferocious in those days—we had to get hold of a Scorpion and burn it, whereupon it was the Lizard that died.

The next thing that we had to be on the look-out for was a Serpent creeping out of his hole. In this emergency we had the choice of three remedies—although 'remedies' is hardly the word to use. However, these remedies are interesting from the comments the Scribe sees fit to add to each of them. The first one directs that ant-fish (dried) be set against the entrance to the Serpent's lair. 'IT WILL NOT CREEP OUT,' added the Scribe. Next he gives us the choice of Natron, which we are to put into the hole. 'IT WILL NOT CREEP OUT,' he adds again to this. But with the third remedy he is even more emphatic still: this is a Garlic-ball which is inserted into the hole, and this time the Scribe confidently adds: 'IT DOES NOT CREEP OUT.'

But squalling children, fleas, lice, wasps, and serpents were not the only annoyances which link us with these Ancients; we also find them in the throes of another scourge that his modern prototype is still engaged in fighting. Albeit we carry on the fight on better—and cleaner—lines:

TO PREVENT THE RODENTS EATING DURRA IN THE GRANARY

Gazelle's dung

Put on the fire in the Granary. Cover the wall and the floor with Mice-excrement and with their urine. That will prevent the durra being eaten.

It would certainly prevent it being eaten by a good many of us.

One last extract from this most human of documents remains to be made:

TO PREVENT THE PIGEON HAWK STEALING

Let a Rod of Acanthus be set up.

The Person says:

'O Horus, the Hawk steals in City and Garden.

'He thirsts after the Garden.

'Fly hither, cook, and eat him.'

Let this be spoken over the Acanthus-rod. Put a Sugar-cake thereon.

HE IT IS WHO PREVENTS THE PIGEON HAWK STEALING.

But a country-side fragrant with sugar-sticks and resounding with prayers is too utterly sentimental for our age. Sugar-sticks have gone down before Scarecrows; the hum of prayers has been drowned in the roar of the charabanc. Not for nothing have fifty centuries of progress and research come and gone.

I

Frontispiece

PORTION OF EBERS PAPYRUS.

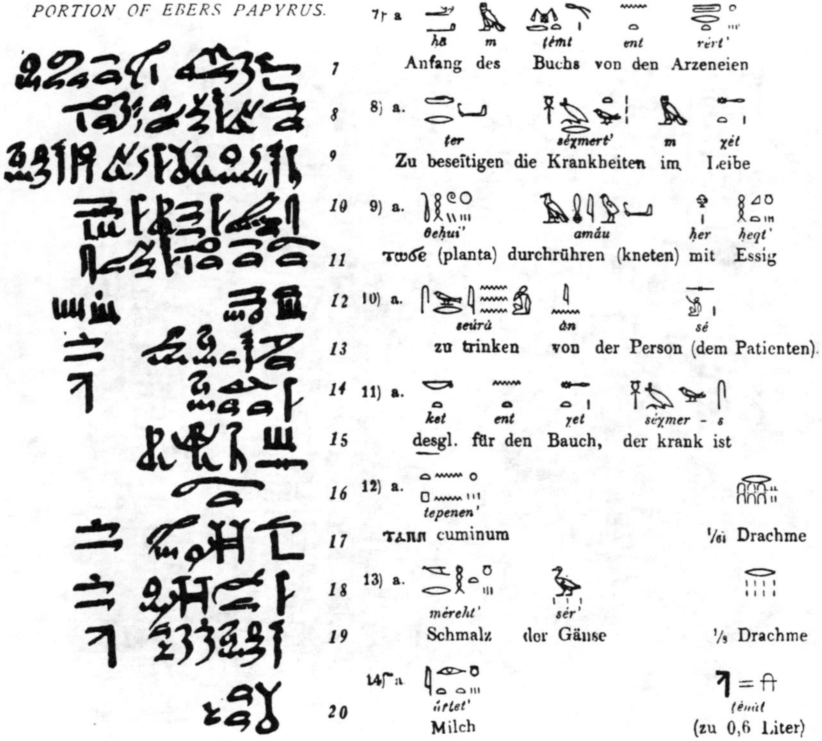

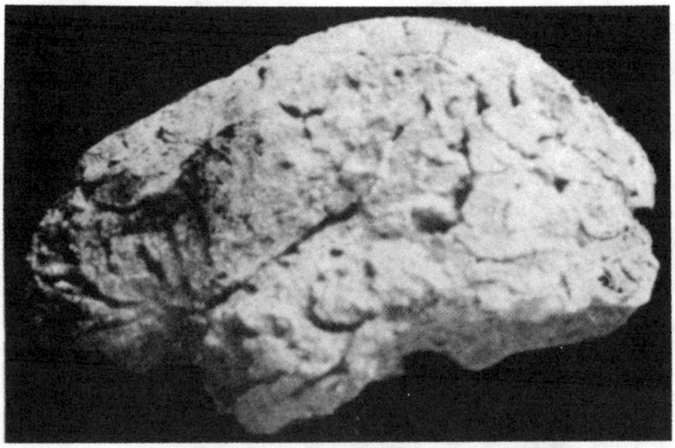

III

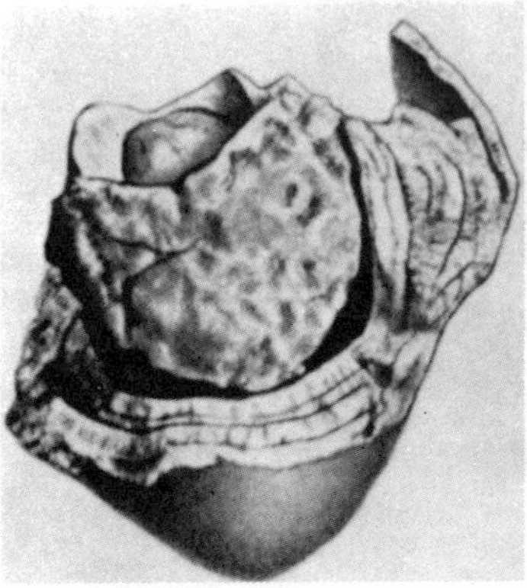

IV

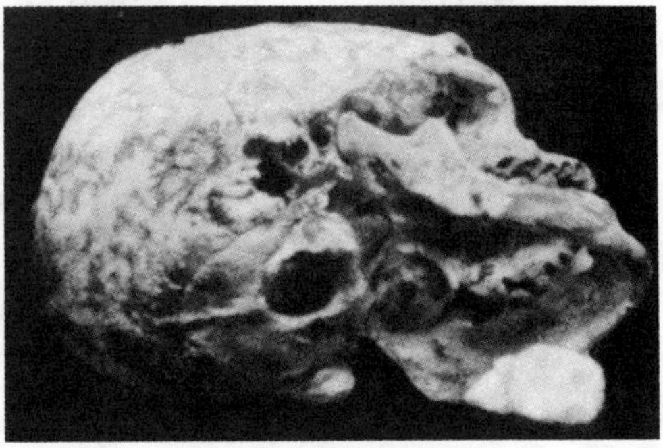

V

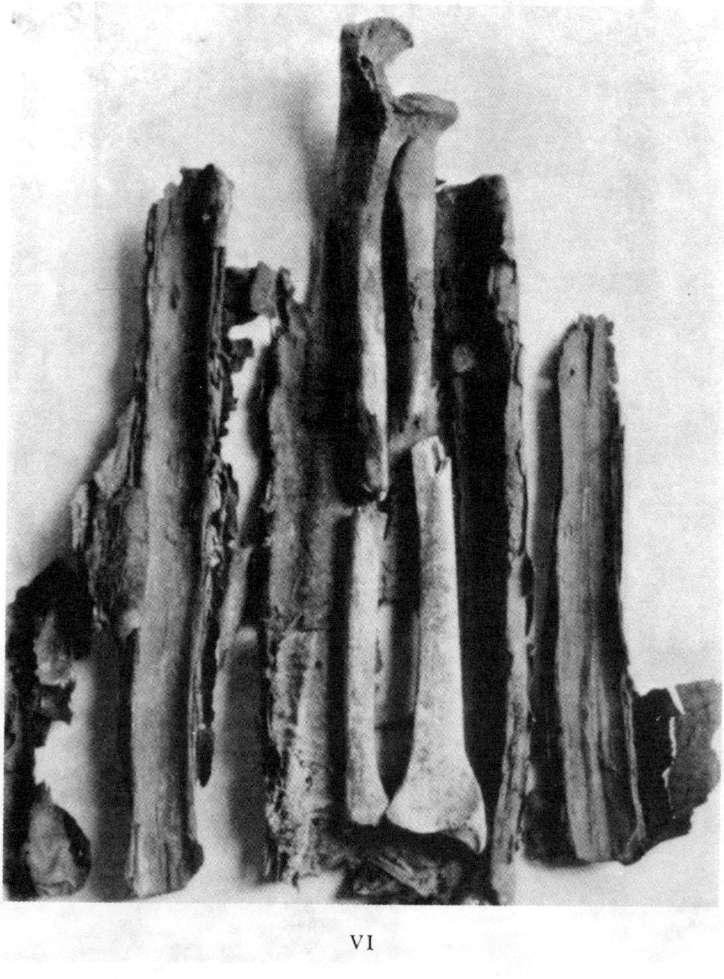

VI

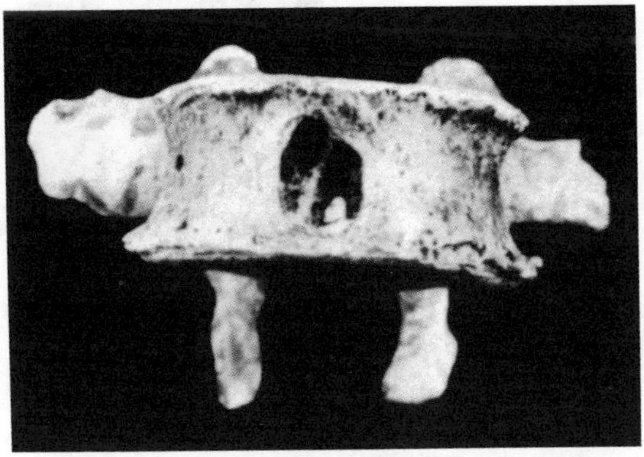

VII

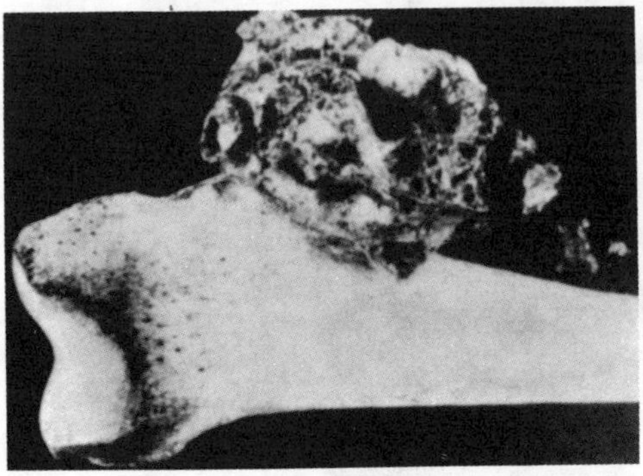

VIII

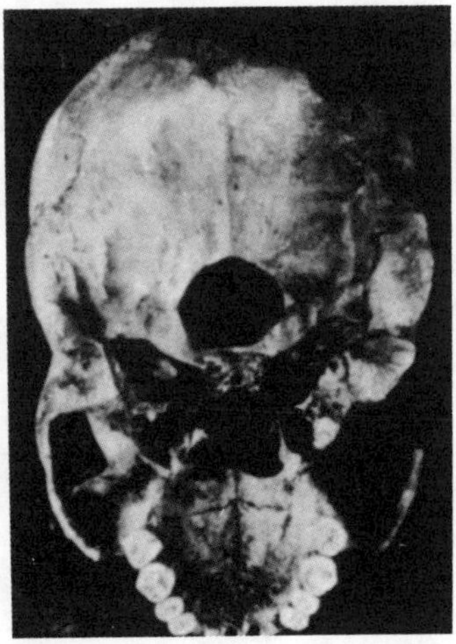

IX

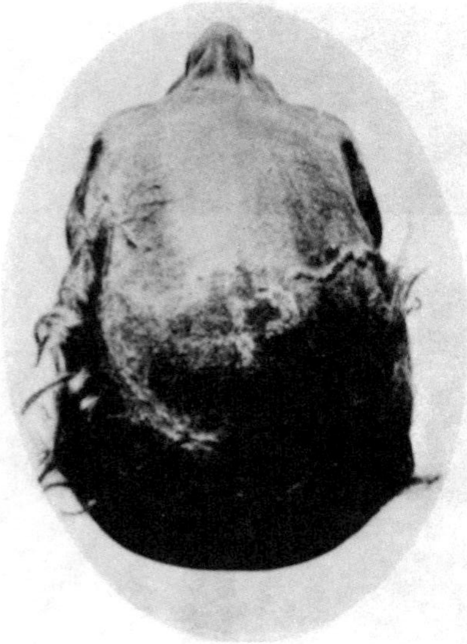
X

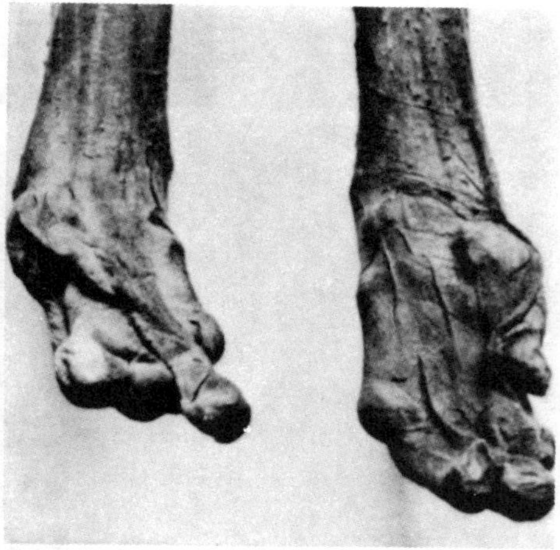
XI

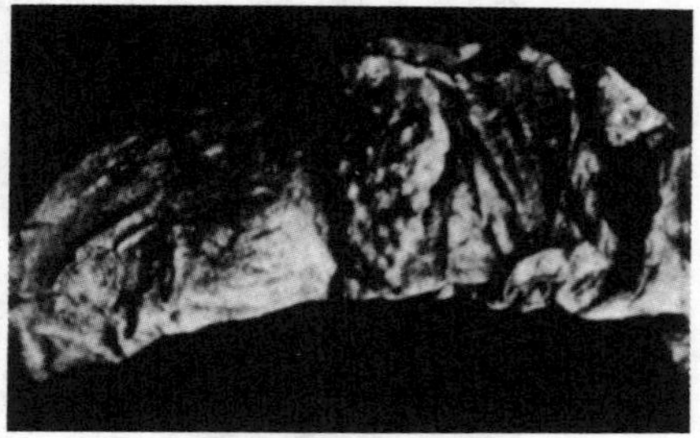
XII

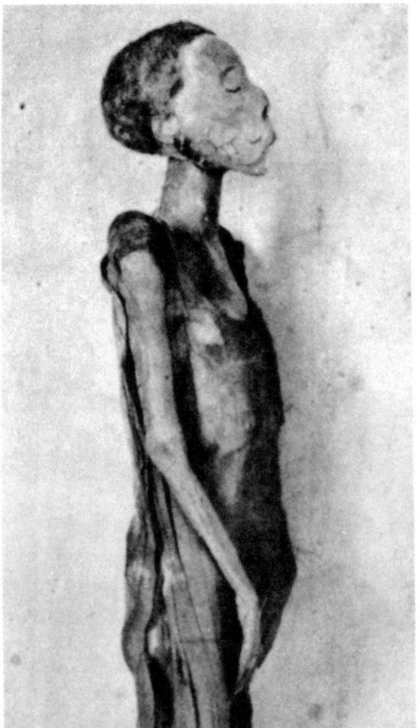

XIII

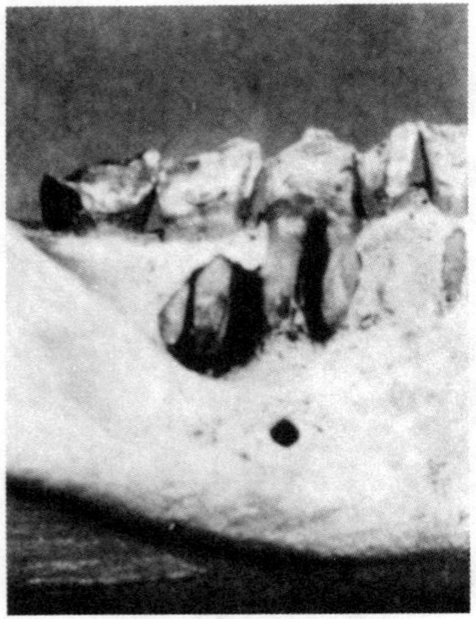

XIV

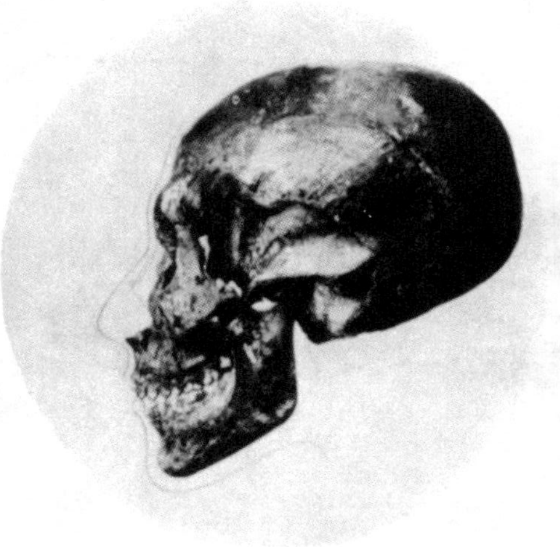

XV

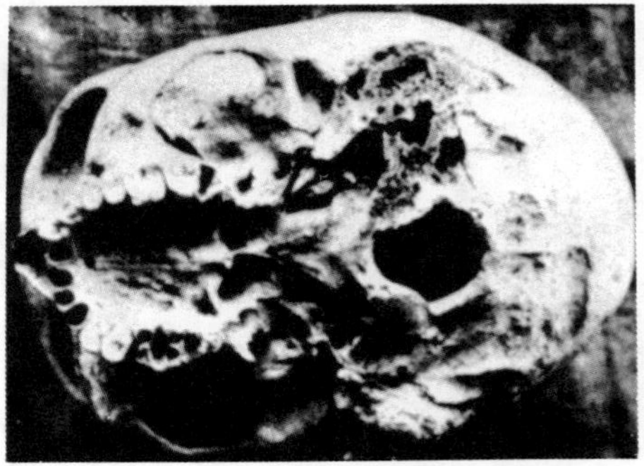

XVI